THE easy diabetes desserts

COOKBOOK

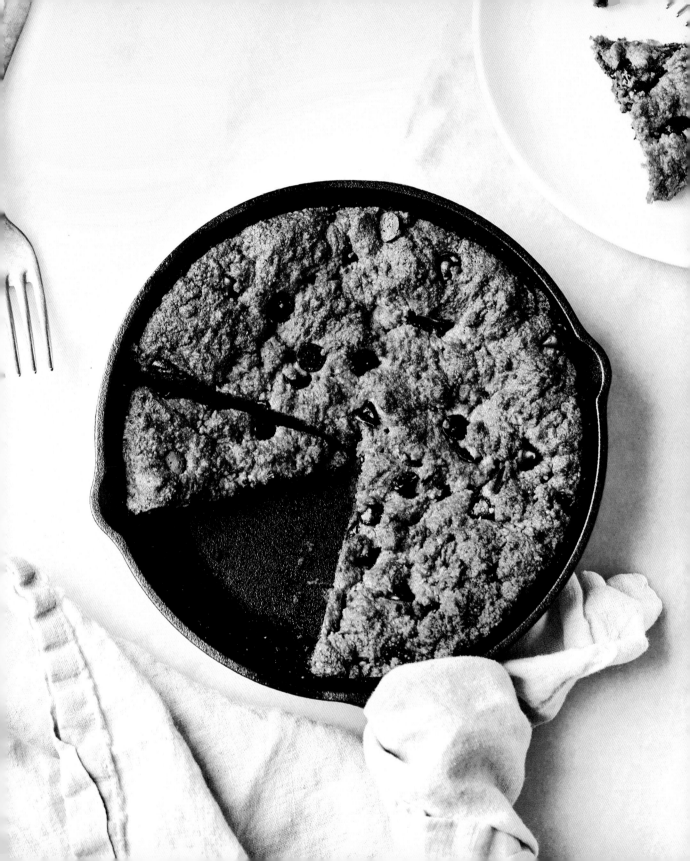

Blood Sugar–Friendly Versions of
Your Favorite Treats

THE *easy* diabetes desserts
COOKBOOK

mary ellen phipps, RDN

author of *The Easy Diabetes Cookbook* and creator of Milk & Honey Nutrition®

PAGE STREET
PUBLISHING CO.

PAGE STREET
PUBLISHING CO.

First published in 2022 by
Page Street Publishing Co.
27 Congress Street, Suite 1511
Salem, MA 01970
www.pagestreetpublishing.com

Distributed by Macmillan, sales in Canada by The Canadian Manda Group.

26   25   24   23   22   1   2   3   4   5

ISBN-13: 978-1-64567-518-1
ISBN-10: 1-64567-518-1

Library of Congress Control Number: 2021937619

Cover and book design by Meg Baskis for Page Street Publishing Co.
Photography by Constance Mariena

Printed and bound in the United States

dedication

To the Milk & Honey Nutrition® community, this book would not have been possible without your support and encouragement. Each and every one of you has played a part in bringing this book to life. I hope you enjoy it.

To my daughters, you are my constant source of motivation and my continual reason for always dreaming big. What a blessing you both are!

And to H, my little diabetes buddy . . . your joy and strength are contagious, and you're going to change the world one day!

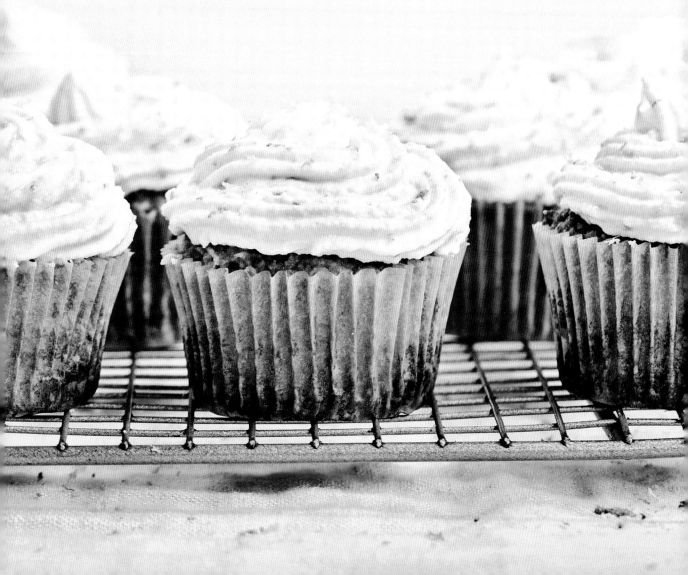

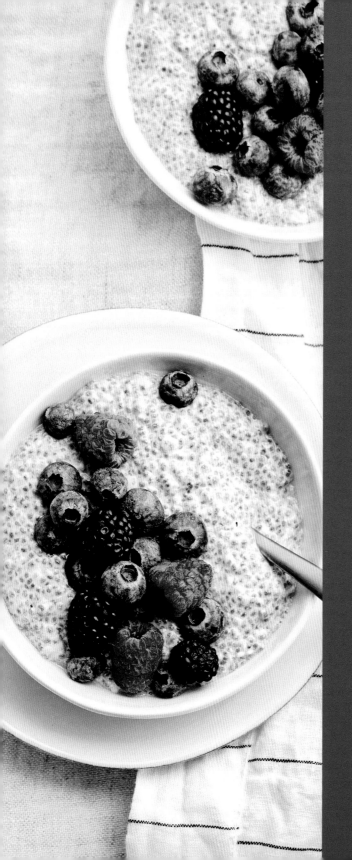

contents

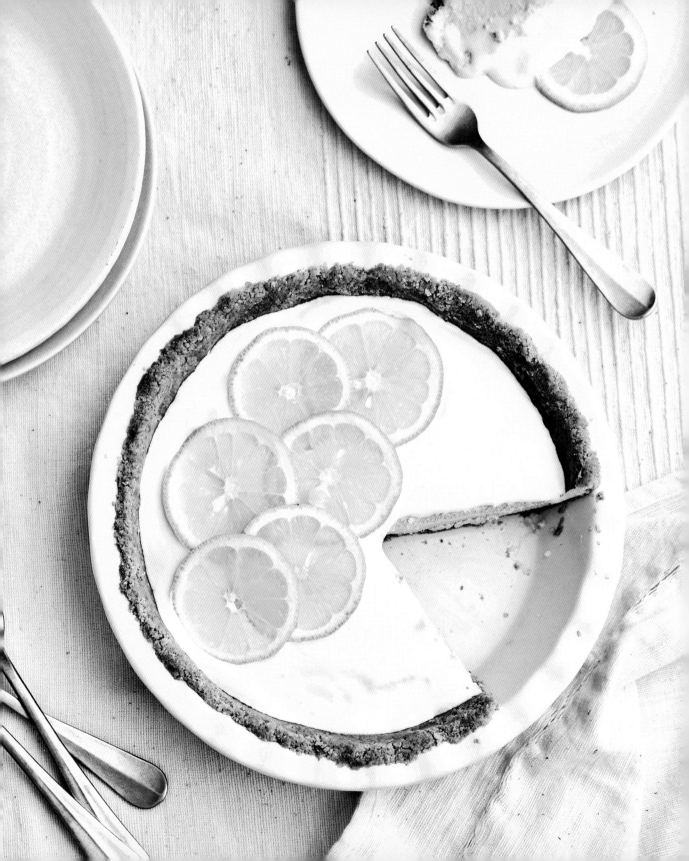

why diabetes doesn't mean an end to dessert

Diabetes and dessert: two words that a lot of people think shouldn't or can't go together. But I'm guessing if you're reading this book, you either hope that's not true or you already know it's not true. As you read through the content and recipes in this book, you're going to learn why diabetes doesn't mean an end to dessert AND how to put that information into practice in the kitchen to make some deliciously blood sugar–friendly desserts.

The beginning of my obsession with desserts . . .

I have been living with diabetes for over 30 years. Back when I was diagnosed as a young child, we didn't have all the different medications and treatment knowledge about diabetes that we do now. So, as a result, what I could and could not eat was very restricted. And as you can imagine, I was not a fan of this.

As I got older and began to notice how the different foods I ate affected my body, I realized I could tweak different recipes and foods to better suit me, my blood sugars, and my diabetes management.

I also had a grandmother who could bake like no other! I'm not kidding. She made the most delicious cakes, cookies, pies, brownies, etc. I could keep going. She had some serious skill in the kitchen. But most of what she made wasn't crafted with blood sugar management in mind . . . until I was diagnosed, that is.

Around the time I was 12, she took me under her wing and showed me the science and art of making desserts . . . and helped me understand how to change a recipe to make it better suit what my body needed, while also still tasting amazing! (The Chocolate Cheesecake with Hazelnut-Spiced Crust [page 60] is based off the recipe she taught me how to make.)

As I grew up, I realized how much I enjoyed making blood sugar–friendly foods taste delicious, and teaching other people how to do that too. So, once I got to college and realized I could make a career out of that, I decided to work towards becoming a registered dietitian.

After earning my bachelor's degree in nutrition science, I completed a graduate school program in public health epidemiology to round out my education. I really learned how to help people understand food better, as well as reduce the amount of anxiety and stress they feel around food.

And quite honestly, that's my goal with this book: to teach you how to conquer the stress and anxiety that you might feel when it comes to diabetes and desserts. I will equip you with the skills to feel confident in the kitchen when baking and cooking, and provide you with some delicious blood sugar–friendly dessert options!

The science behind diabetes and dessert

When you look at a typical cake, cookie, or pie recipe, there's usually a lot of sugar and saturated fat, and not a whole lot of fiber and protein. In other words: a perfect formula for a blood sugar spike. That's because fat, fiber, and protein slow down the digestion process. Without those, digestion happens quickly and blood sugars can rise really fast.

Fat, fiber, and protein all act like buffers when it comes to blood sugars. If you were to eat just carbohydrates, or just sugar, your blood sugar would rise really quickly. But, if you eat the same amount of sugar combined with some fat, fiber, and/or protein, they will rise more slowly and we can avoid rapid blood sugar spikes.

So, what if we knew how to reduce the sugar content, swap those saturated fats out for plant-based fats, and up the protein and fiber content of these dessert recipes, while keeping our desserts tasting delicious at the same time? That would be pretty amazing, right?!

Well, that's exactly what you'll find in the 60 delicious blood sugar–friendly dessert recipes in this book. They are lower in sugar, and higher in:

- Plant-based fats
- Fiber
- Protein

As I mention above, when foods are high in fat, fiber, and/or protein, it takes our bodies longer to digest the food. This is a good thing! The slower the digestion process, the slower (and more consistent) the nutrient absorption . . . including the sugar that's also in the recipe.

By choosing ingredients that are higher in plant-based fats, fiber, and protein, we're giving our bodies the additional nutrients they need to slowly digest the sugar that's in the dessert recipe and thus prevent potential rapid blood sugar spikes. And this is what makes these recipes perfectly suited for people with diabetes!

Foolproof Strategies for Delicious Blood Sugar–Friendly Desserts

Now that we've covered what we're aiming for when making blood sugar–friendly desserts . . .

- Less sugar
- More plant-based fat
- More fiber
- More protein
- Amazing taste!

. . . let's take a look at my five go-to strategies for accomplishing these goals in a recipe. You'll see these used throughout the recipes in this book.

1. Cut the sugar: You can actually take a typical dessert recipe and cut the amount of sugar called for by up to half and still make a delicious dessert that tastes amazing!

2. Add beans or lentils: Ok, I know it sounds weird, but when you mash up cooked beans or lentils, they have a pretty similar texture to cookie dough! By adding these to a recipe, we're increasing the fiber and protein content. Remember, fiber and protein both help to promote stable blood sugars after you eat. And don't worry, we'll be sure to mask the flavor of them with other delicious flavor enhancers like cinnamon and vanilla extract, so you won't even be able to taste that they're in there.

3. Swap the fat: Swapping out butter for something like avocado, avocado oil, or even pumpkin puree will reduce the amount of saturated fat in a recipe. And we know from years of research that people with diabetes should limit how much saturated fat they consume.

4. Play around with flours: This is the strategy you'll notice happening most often in this cookbook. Nut-based flours like almond flour, walnut flour, and coconut flour have fewer carbohydrates and more plant-based fat than traditional refined flours. Both lowering the carbohydrate count and increasing plant-based fat are great for promoting stable blood sugars. And don't forget to check out the substitution chart on page 16 if you don't have one of the flours listed in a recipe.

5. Grab the yogurt: Both plain yogurt and plain Greek yogurt work to enhance the flavor of a recipe and increase the protein content without adding unnecessary sugar. Yogurt can be subbed in for a fat source or used as a wet ingredient to achieve the right consistency in a dough or batter.

And remember, a diabetes-friendly dessert doesn't automatically mean a "diet" or "light" dessert. Or at least, it shouldn't. Sometimes we want a dessert that is equally rich and decadent, but just a bit easier on blood sugars. And that's what this book is for: to help you celebrate all of life's amazing occasions, whether it's a birthday with Funfetti® Birthday Cake (page 66) or just a simple weekday morning with some Classic Blueberry Banana Bread (page 87).

A Closer Look at Ingredients

Whether you're reading through this book trying to understand why I use certain ingredients, or trying to make another recipe at home more blood sugar friendly, I want you to understand how these ingredients work to balance blood sugars and increase your confidence for blood sugar–friendly baking! Specifically, I want to show you how picking the right flours and sweeteners can make all the difference in how your blood sugars respond to a dessert, and what to do if you don't have an ingredient on hand.

What Types of Sugar and Sweeteners Are Best?

It's only fitting that in a book all about blood sugar–friendly desserts, we talk about what kinds of sweeteners we'll be using, right? But, there is definitely more to this conversation than what is best for blood sugars. We need to balance what is best for blood sugars and managing diabetes with a recipe that still tastes amazing and is simple to make.

So, what kinds of sweeteners exist that are blood sugar friendly, still taste delicious, are easy to find at your local grocery store, and are universally appealing?

In planning out the recipes for this book, I wanted to make sure I was using sweeteners that most people have easy access to and that aren't super expensive. I also purposely chose not to use non-nutritive sweeteners or artificial sweeteners in any of the recipes in this book, and I'll explain more about why I did that in a bit.

You'll see in the recipes that follow that I use the following sweeteners most often: coconut sugar, table sugar, maple syrup, honey, and agave nectar. Which one I choose to use is dependent on a few factors:

- Do I want to use a wet sweetener or a dry sweetener?
- What other ingredients am I using in the recipe?
- How sweet tasting do we want it to be?
- What color do we want the final product to be?

	Grams of sugar per tbsp	Primary form of sugar	Are other beneficial nutrients present?	Does it have a lower glycemic index than table sugar?
Table sugar	12	Sucrose	No	N/A
Coconut sugar	12	Sucrose	Yes: iron, zinc, calcium, potassium, antioxidants, inulin (a form of fiber)	Yes, because of the fiber that is present, though the difference is small
Maple syrup	12	Sucrose	Yes: manganese, zinc, and other antioxidants	Yes
Honey	17	Fructose and glucose	Yes: many vitamins, minerals, and antioxidants, as well as possible functional medicine properties	Yes
Agave nectar	16	Fructose	Yes: small amounts of B vitamins	Yes

All of these sweeteners contribute sugar to a recipe. And that's okay. We are balancing out those grams of sugar with other fat, fiber, and protein-rich ingredients.

You'll notice my choice of sweetener doesn't really have anything to do with how much sugar it contains. That's because I know what matters more is the overall amount of sweetener we're using and the other ingredients present in the recipe.

As you can see in the table above, there are small differences in the types of sugars and their different properties. But these small differences aren't really all that relevant when we take a step back and remember they are all still forms of sugar. This is why the type of sweetener I have chosen in each recipe in this book is actually based on the desired taste and flavor, and is used in moderation and balance with other ingredients.

What About Non-nutritive Sweeteners or Artificial Sweeteners?

Non-nutritive sweeteners contain few to no calories or nutrients. They can be made in a lab, or produced from plants or herbs, or even sugar itself. They are much sweeter than actual sugar, so you don't need to use as much to sweeten recipes. Some naturally derived non-nutritive sweeteners are excellent tools to help manage blood sugars. So, why did I choose not to use them in this book?

Well, quite simply, I want everyone to enjoy every recipe in this book. I want the ingredients to be things you have easy access to. And I want the ingredients used to be universally appealing. Non-nutritive sweeteners (both natural and artificial) can be a polarizing topic, and I didn't want one being listed in the recipe to be a reason for someone not to try it.

If you have one you love, however, and know how to make proper substitutions (you can check out some options on page 16 in the substitution chart), I say go for it. Just keep in mind the carbohydrate and sugar content of your finished product will be different than what is listed under the recipe.

Working with Blood Sugar–Friendly Flours

Baked goods like cookies, brownies, pies, and more are often foods people with diabetes think they're not allowed to eat. But, as you've hopefully gathered by now, that is not true! We just need to pay attention to what we're putting into our favorite sweet treats.

All of the recipes in this book prioritize increasing some combination of fat, fiber, and protein in the final dessert product. And there are many different ways to achieve this. One of those ways is by using more blood sugar–friendly flours. Blood sugar–friendly flours (examples below) will have fewer carbohydrates and more fat and protein than traditional all-purpose wheat or rice flours. All-purpose flour does have some protein, but that's about it. So, in our blood sugar–friendly baking, we're going to opt for flours with fewer carbohydrates, and more protein and fat.

Now, there are a TON of flour options available at your local grocery store, and we won't dive into all of those. But I do want to take a minute and discuss the flours you will see used most frequently in this book.

I've been baking and creating dessert recipes with these four flours for years, and time and time again they prove that you can enjoy a blood sugar–friendly dessert that is equally (or even more!) delicious and satisfying!

ALMOND FLOUR

Almond flour is probably the most well-known and widely used grain-free flour on the market, and really started to gain mainstream popularity 10 to 15 years ago when eating gluten free and/or Paleo started to become more popular.

Now, as a dietitian, I do feel like it's my job to stop here and remind you that eating gluten free is not inherently better for you unless you have a gluten intolerance or have celiac disease. The reason I prefer almond flour in recipes is not because it is gluten free, but rather because of its macronutrient makeup (carbs, fat, and protein).

You can see the chart on page 16 to compare, but almond flour has dramatically fewer carbohydrates, more fiber, more protein, and more fat compared to all-purpose flour.

When used by itself, almond flour can often result in a crumbly mess, though, so we combine it with another flour like oat flour or tapioca flour/starch to create a cohesive baked good.

OAT FLOUR (A.K.A. GROUND-UP OATS)

Oat flour has a comparable amount of carbohydrates to all-purpose flour, but has more fiber and fat, making it a bit more blood sugar friendly. It also pairs well with almond flour in baked goods to create a palatable texture.

A little kitchen hack that will save you a lot of money at the grocery store and help with many of the recipes in this book is making your own oat flour at home. All you have to do is grind up rolled oats! And that's it. That's oat flour.

COCONUT FLOUR

Coconut flour is used for its high protein and fiber content and I love to use it in no-bake recipes to absorb liquid and help us achieve the desired consistency. It also pairs nicely with almond flour to help baked goods hold together.

One small note that's important to remember about coconut flour is that it should never be substituted cup for cup for other flours. See the substitution chart on page 16 for tips, but just remember coconut flour absorbs far more liquid than other flours, so subbing it into a recipe cup for cup will usually result in very dry, crumbly desserts.

TAPIOCA FLOUR

A quick look at the chart below and you'll see tapioca flour isn't exactly blood sugar friendly. There's no fat, fiber, or protein anywhere in sight. But, I sometimes like to use a small amount combined with larger quantities of our other blood sugar–friendly flours to achieve a more desirable texture than just using almond, coconut, or oat flour on their own.

100 g of . . .	All-purpose wheat-based flour	Almond flour	Oat flour	Coconut flour	Tapioca flour/starch
Total Carbohydrates	77.3 g	21.3 g	73.3 g	60 g	87.5 g
Fiber	2.7 g	7.1 g	10 g	33.3 g	0 g
Protein	10.9 g	21.4 g	13.33 g	20 g	0 g
Fat	1.5 g	53.6 g	6.7 g	13.3 g	0 g
Can it be consumed raw?	No	Yes	Yes	Yes	Sometimes

When You Don't Have an Ingredient on Hand

Don't have an ingredient on hand? No worries! Try any of the substitutions listed below:

The recipe calls for . . .	but you can also sub in . . .
Almond flour	Coconut flour can work, but you only need one third of the amount of coconut flour (1 cup [95 g] of almond flour = ⅓ cup [40 g] of coconut flour). You can also try equal quantities (to the amount of almond flour called for in your recipe) of another nut-based flour.
Oat flour	You don't need to buy oat flour, but can actually make your own—just grind up oats! Other options: wheat flour (only for baked/cooked goods; wheat flour should not be consumed raw), gluten-free flour blend, sorghum flour.
Coconut flour	Almond flour is the best option here. Remember, ⅓ cup (40 g) of coconut flour = 1 cup (95 g) of almond flour.
Tapioca flour	Arrowroot powder, cornstarch, or potato starch
Xanthan gum	Guar gum, ground chia seeds, or ground flax seeds
Nut butter	Sunflower seed butter, pumpkin seed butter, or coconut butter
Coconut oil	Butter or ghee will work for baked goods. Olive oil or avocado oil will work for dishes that aren't being baked.

Oil (liquid at room temperature)	Most oils can be subbed in and out for each other. Just keep in mind the different flavors that may be present.
Milk	Dairy-free milk, like almond milk, plain yogurt, plain kefir, or sour cream
Yogurt	Plain Greek yogurt or plain kefir. And some baked goods like cookies or bars can use equal quantities of pumpkin puree instead of yogurt.
Eggs	¼ cup of any of the following: unsweetened applesauce, plain yogurt, silken tofu, mashed banana You can also make a chia or flax egg: Combine 1 tablespoon (10 g) of ground chia or flax seeds with 3 tablespoons (45 ml) of water in a small bowl and let it sit for a few minutes until it is thick and gelatinous. Then add the mixture to your recipe.
Maple syrup	An equal quantity of agave nectar, honey, sugar-free syrup, molasses, or corn syrup will give you the same texture, though the flavors will be different depending on the sweetener you choose.
Coconut sugar or table sugar	An equal quantity of any granulated sweetener will work, unless you are using a product (like an alternative sweetener) that offers a conversion chart with different amounts. If this is the case, coconut sugar is considered the same as table sugar when determining substitution quantities for this type of product.
Vanilla extract	Almond extract is my favorite substitute for vanilla extract. It adds a different flavor but is equally tasty in baked goods.

Symbols/Categories

As you go through the recipes in this cookbook, you'll see the descriptors below on various recipes. These are meant to help you easily see what different nutritional characteristics each recipe has.

Gluten-Free: All ingredients used in the recipe are naturally gluten free (also remember you can substitute gluten-free oats for traditional oats in any recipe!).

No Added Sugar: All sugar in the recipe comes from naturally occurring sources like fruit, milk, and flours.

Dairy-Free: No dairy ingredients are used in the recipe.

High Protein: One serving of the recipe contains 5 grams or more of protein.

High Fiber: One serving of the recipe contains 5 grams or more of fiber.

Quick & Simple: The recipe takes less than 1 hour to make from start to finish.

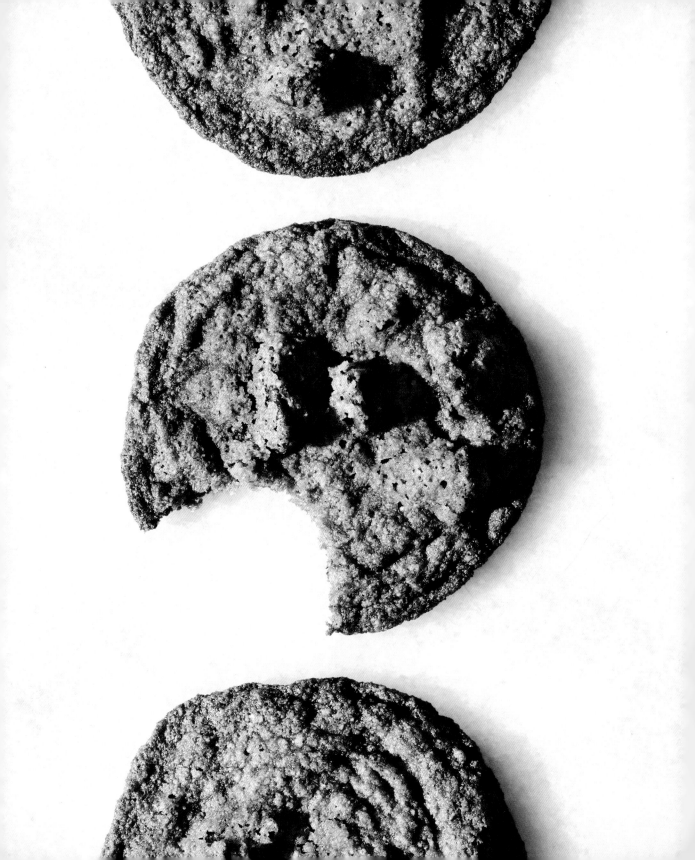

not your average cookies

Cookies. They're everyone's favorite. In fact, I don't think I've ever met a person who *doesn't* like cookies. That feeling of biting into a warm cookie with the perfect texture just can't be beat!

Often, people with diabetes feel like they can't enjoy a cookie, or the so-called "healthy" cookies they're told to choose instead are bland and taste like poorly sweetened cardboard. But, what if I told you there was a way to make blood sugar–friendly and completely balanced cookies that also taste just as good as (and sometimes better than!) traditional cookies? You'd be pretty excited, right?

The three ingredients we want to try to modify or adjust when crafting a more blood sugar–friendly cookie recipe are:

- **Flour:** We will choose flours that have fewer carbohydrates, and more protein and fat, than traditional all-purpose flour.
- **Sugar:** We'll cut back on the amount of sweetener used because oftentimes, you just don't need that much to get a tasty dessert you'll enjoy!
- **Butter:** In many of the recipes we'll choose things like avocado oil or coconut oil for a plant-based alternative.

So, all of the cookie recipes you'll see in this section, from the Zesty Orange Sugar Cookies (page 27) to the Pecan Praline Cookies (page 36), have a blood sugar–friendly twist on one or more of those three ingredients. I know you're going to love all of them!

crunchy hazelnut chocolate chip cookies

These cookies use one of my favorite tricks for making delicious blood sugar–friendly cookies: ground-up nuts instead of flour! The flavor of the hazelnuts and walnuts combined is just perfection. Oh, and there's only 11 grams of carbohydrates per cookie (and they're big, too!).

gluten-free | yield: 24 cookies

1½ cups (176 g) walnut halves

1½ cups (173 g) chopped hazelnuts

⅓ cup (76 g) unsalted butter, softened and cut into small cubes

⅓ cup (80 ml) maple syrup

¼ tsp salt

½ tsp baking soda

2 tsp (10 ml) vanilla extract

1 tsp almond extract

½ cup (84 g) chocolate chips

TIP: You don't have to refrigerate your dough. You can go ahead and bake the cookies right after you mix up the dough, but they will spread out more on the pan while baking, so make sure to allow more room on the pan, 2½ to 3 inches (6 to 8 cm) between cookies.

Nutrition Info (Serving size: 1 cookie): Calories: 148, Total Fat: 12 g, Saturated Fat: 3 g, Total Carbohydrates: 8.5 g, Sugar: 6 g, Fiber: 1 g, Sodium: 51 mg, Protein: 2 g

Preheat your oven to 350°F (177°C). Line a baking sheet with parchment paper and set it aside.

In a food processor, process your walnut halves and chopped hazelnuts until a powder forms. As soon as you see that the mixture resembles a powder, stop the food processor (do not over-process them, as this will lead to some of the oil separating from the nuts, which will make it difficult for the cookies to set).

Add in the butter and pulse the mixture in the food processor until it's well combined. Next, add the maple syrup, salt, baking soda, vanilla extract, and almond extract to the food processor.

Process the mixture for 20 to 30 seconds, until a dough forms. Again, be careful not to over-process the dough.

Carefully remove the blade from the food processor and stir in the chocolate chips by hand.

Place your dough in the refrigerator for 1 hour or let it sit in the freezer for 20 minutes before trying to scoop the dough onto your pan.

Using a small cookie scoop or a tablespoon, scoop the dough into balls and place them about 1½ inches (4 cm) apart from each other on your parchment-lined baking sheet. Gently press the dough balls down with a fork to flatten them into circles.

Bake the cookies for 18 to 20 minutes, or until the edges of the cookies are set and the tops start to turn golden brown. Remove the cookies from the oven and let them cool for 4 to 5 minutes before carefully transferring them to a wire rack to finish cooling completely.

Store your cookies in an airtight container with a paper towel underneath the cookies in the bottom of the container to absorb any liquid/natural oils. Eat within 48 hours or freeze.

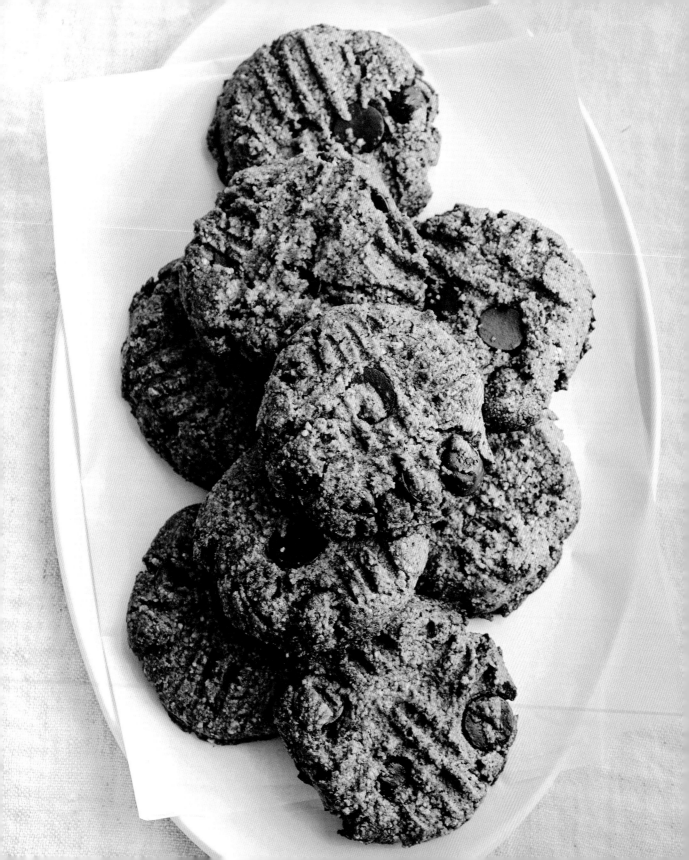

oatmeal raisin chai spice cookies

You might hear the word "raisin" and think these cookies are immediately off-limits if you're trying to balance blood sugars. But that's not true! It's a common myth that people with diabetes can't eat dried fruit. It's all about how much you're eating and what you're eating it with. By using a combination of almond flour and oats for the base of these cookies, we're balancing things out for a delicious blood sugar–friendly cookie!

dairy-free | high protein | quick & simple | yield: 10 cookies

1¼ cups (113 g) rolled oats

1 cup (95 g) almond flour

1 tsp baking powder

½ tsp baking soda

1 tsp ground cinnamon

1 tsp chai spice blend

¼ tsp salt

¼ cup (50 g) granulated sugar

¼ cup (60 ml) oil

1 large egg, beaten

2 tsp (10 ml) vanilla extract

½ cup (120 ml) unsweetened applesauce

½ cup (73 g) raisins, not packed

First, preheat your oven to 375°F (191°C). Line a baking sheet with parchment paper and set it aside.

In a medium-sized bowl, combine the oats, almond flour, baking powder, baking soda, cinnamon, chai spice blend, salt, and sugar. Whisk them all lightly together to combine. Set the dry mixture aside.

In a separate large bowl, combine the oil, egg, vanilla extract, and applesauce. Whisk the wet mixture together thoroughly until combined. Now, add the dry ingredients to the wet ingredients and stir with a rubber spatula just until combined. Add the raisins to the bowl and mix it all together until combined.

Using a large cookie scoop (or ice cream scoop), scoop the dough onto the prepared baking sheet, making sure the scoops are 1 to 2 inches (2.5 to 5 cm) apart. Bake for 18 to 20 minutes, or until the tops are golden brown and the cookies have begun to set.

Remove the cookies from the oven and let them cool for 5 to 10 minutes, then transfer them to a cooling rack to finish cooling.

Store your cookies in an airtight container in the refrigerator for 5 to 7 days, or freeze them for up to 3 months.

TIP: If you can't find a chai spice blend at your local store, you can make your own by mixing together ⅛ teaspoon of cardamom, ⅛ teaspoon of allspice, ⅛ teaspoon of nutmeg, ⅛ teaspoon of ground cloves, ½ teaspoon of ground cinnamon, and ½ teaspoon of ground ginger.

Nutrition Info (Serving size: 1 cookie):
Calories: 203, Total Fat: 11 g, Saturated Fat: 1 g, Total Carbohydrates: 22 g, Sugar: 11 g, Fiber: 3 g, Sodium: 131 mg, Protein: 5 g

white chocolate macadamia nut cookie cups

Get ready for a classically soft and fluffy white chocolate cookie, but made in a muffin cup! These cookie cups are made with nutrient-rich ingredients and about half the amount of sugar as normal cookies. So grab one and leave the blood sugar worries behind!

quick & simple | yield: 12 cookie cups

¼ cup (60 ml) plain whole milk Greek yogurt

¼ cup (57 g) unsalted butter, softened

½ cup (100 g) cane sugar

2 large eggs

1 tsp vanilla extract

1½ cups (135 g) rolled oats, ground

¼ tsp baking soda

¼ tsp baking powder

⅓ cup (45 g) chopped macadamia nuts

⅓ cup (56 g) white chocolate chips

Preheat your oven to 350°F (177°C). Line the wells of a muffin tin and set it aside.

In the bowl of a stand mixer, combine the Greek yogurt and softened butter and mix for 1 to 2 minutes on medium speed until well combined. Then, add in the cane sugar, and mix until combined. Next, we'll add in the eggs and vanilla extract and mix again until combined.

In a separate bowl, combine the ground oats, baking soda, and baking powder and whisk gently to combine. Add the dry mixture to the bowl with the yogurt/butter mixture. Mix on medium speed until a dough forms, or for about 1 minute.

Remove the bowl from the mixer and mix the macadamia nuts and white chocolate chips in by hand. Using a cookie scoop, drop the dough into the wells of the prepared muffin tin.

Bake for 20 to 22 minutes, or until the tops begin to turn golden brown.

Remove the cookie cups from the oven and let them cool completely before removing them from the muffin tin.

Store your cookie cups in an airtight container on the counter for up to 5 days, in the refrigerator for up to 10 days, or in the freezer for up to 6 months.

TIP: If you have them, I recommend using silicone muffin liners!

Nutrition Info (Serving size: 1 cookie cup): Calories: 179, Total Fat: 10 g, Saturated Fat: 5 g, Total Carbohydrates: 20 g, Sugar: 13 g, Fiber: 1 g, Sodium: 50 mg, Protein: 4 g

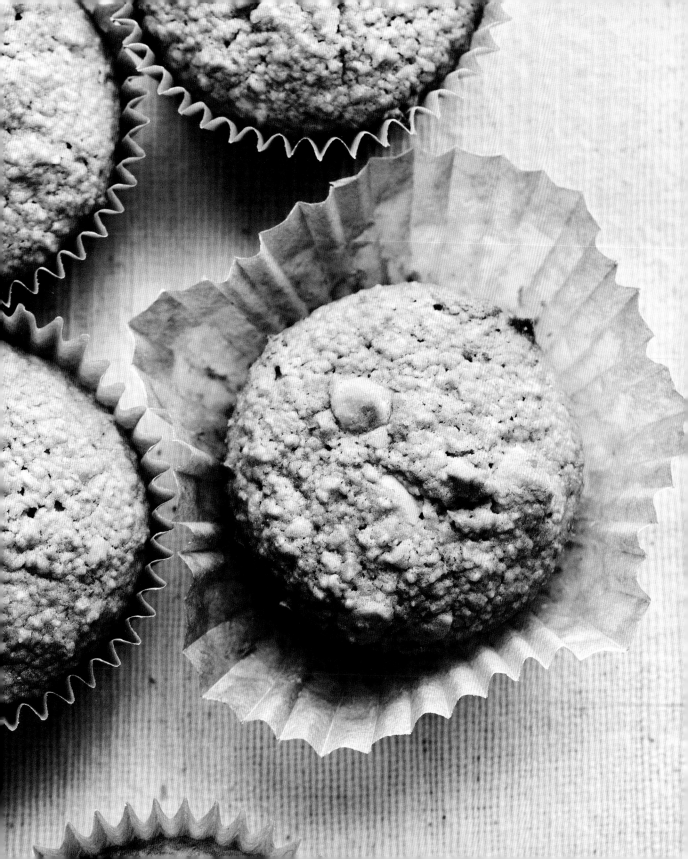

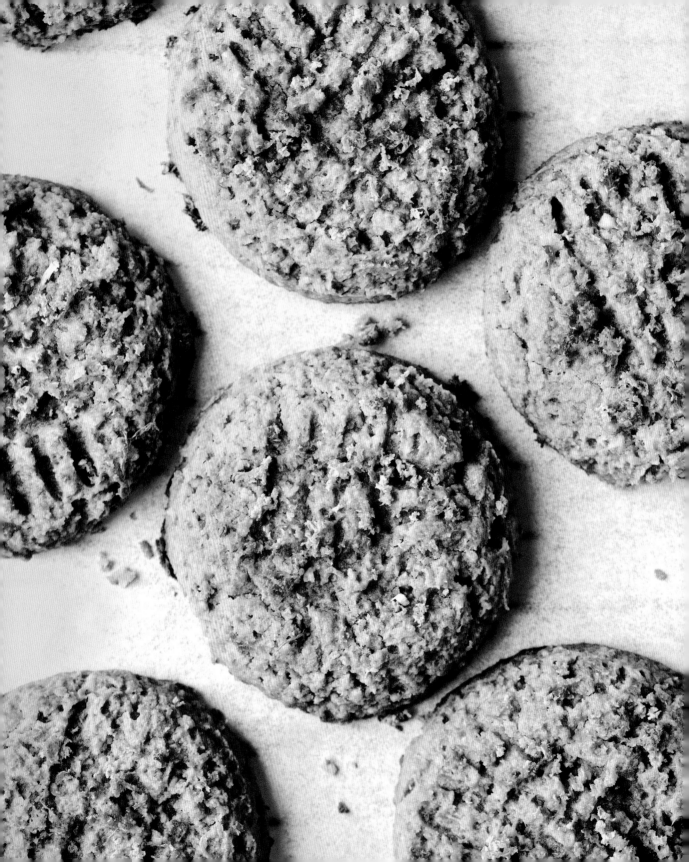

zesty orange sugar cookies

Now, I know the secret ingredient in these delicious Zesty Orange Sugar Cookies might catch you off guard, but don't knock it 'til you've tried it! By adding chickpeas to this batter, we're increasing the protein and fiber, and also adding the blood sugar–stabilizing power of beans. Some research shows that eating beans can help promote stable blood sugars for up to 24 hours after you eat them!

dairy-free | yield: 12 cookies

1 cup (90 g) rolled oats

1 (15-oz [425-g]) can low-sodium chickpeas, rinsed and drained

¼ cup (60 ml) oil

1½ tsp (8 ml) vanilla extract

¼ tsp baking soda

1 tsp baking powder

¼ tsp salt

¼ cup (60 ml) agave nectar

3 tbsp (45 ml) orange juice

½ tbsp (2 g) orange zest, divided

Preheat your oven to 350°F (177°C). Line a baking sheet with parchment paper and set it aside.

In the bowl of a large food processor, place the oats, chickpeas, oil, vanilla extract, baking soda, baking powder, salt, agave, orange juice, and ¼ tablespoon (1 g) of orange zest. Process on high for about a minute, until your batter is a smooth consistency. You may need to stop the food processor once or twice and scrape down the sides as it blends together.

Once the batter is one consistency, remove the blade. Place the dough in the refrigerator for at least 2 hours to firm up.

Once chilled, use an ice cream scoop to drop the batter about 2 inches (5 cm) apart onto the prepared baking sheet. Using a fork, gently press the dough scoops flat. Sprinkle the dough with the remaining ¼ tablespoon (1 g) of orange zest.

Place the pan in the oven and bake for 20 minutes, until they're set and the tops are golden brown.

Remove the pan from the oven and let the cookies sit on the pan for 5 minutes. Then transfer the cookies to a cooling rack.

Store in an airtight container for up to 3 days on the counter, up to 2 weeks in the refrigerator, or up to 6 months in the freezer.

TIPS: Want to turn these into lemon or lime cookies? Just swap out the orange zest for lemon or lime zest!

These cookies won't change shape much when you bake them, so if you want perfect round circles, make sure to smooth out those edges before they go in the oven.

Nutrition Info (Serving size: 1 cookie): Calories: 115, Total Fat: 6 g, Saturated Fat: <1 g, Total Carbohydrates: 16 g, Sugar: 6 g, Fiber: 2 g, Sodium: 133 mg, Protein: 2 g

chewy chocolate cookies

These cookies are deliciously rich and chocolatey. With only 17 grams of carbohydrates in each cookie, they're the perfect after-dinner sweet treat that also happens to offer some additional protein as well. These cookies would also make the perfect "bread" for a homemade ice cream sandwich with some low-sugar ice cream!

dairy-free | yield: 24 cookies

1½ cups (150 g) coconut sugar

½ cup (108 ml) refined coconut oil, softened

1 tsp vanilla extract

½ tsp almond extract

2 large eggs

1½ cups (143 g) almond flour

½ cup (60 g) tapioca flour

½ cup (44 g) unsweetened cocoa powder

1 tsp cream of tartar

½ tsp baking soda

¼ tsp salt

Preheat your oven to 400°F (204°C) and line a baking sheet with parchment paper. Set it aside.

In a large bowl, beat the coconut sugar and coconut oil until thoroughly mixed. Add the vanilla extract, almond extract, and eggs to the bowl, and beat until combined.

Add the almond flour, tapioca flour, cocoa powder, cream of tartar, baking soda, and salt. Beat until well combined. Chill the dough in the refrigerator for at least 2 hours.

Use a cookie scoop or your hands to form the dough into 1 inch (2.5 cm) balls. Place the dough balls 2 inches (5 cm) apart on the prepared baking sheet. Press the balls down flat gently with your hand. Bake the cookies for 10 minutes, or until the edges appear set and slightly crispy.

Remove the cookies from the oven and let them cool on the parchment paper until they are no longer hot. Letting them cool fully gives the edges of the cookies time to crisp up.

Store your cookies in a sealed container on the counter for 5 to 7 days, or freeze for up to 6 months.

TIP: Once you store these in a sealed container, they may lose some of their crispiness on the edges. But you can reheat them in an air fryer or toaster oven for a minute or two to help the edges crisp back up.

Nutrition Info (Serving size: 1 cookie): Calories: 141, Total Fat: 8 g, Saturated Fat: 4.5 g, Total Carbohydrates: 17 g, Sugar: 12 g, Fiber: 1 g, Sodium: 57 mg, Protein: 3 g

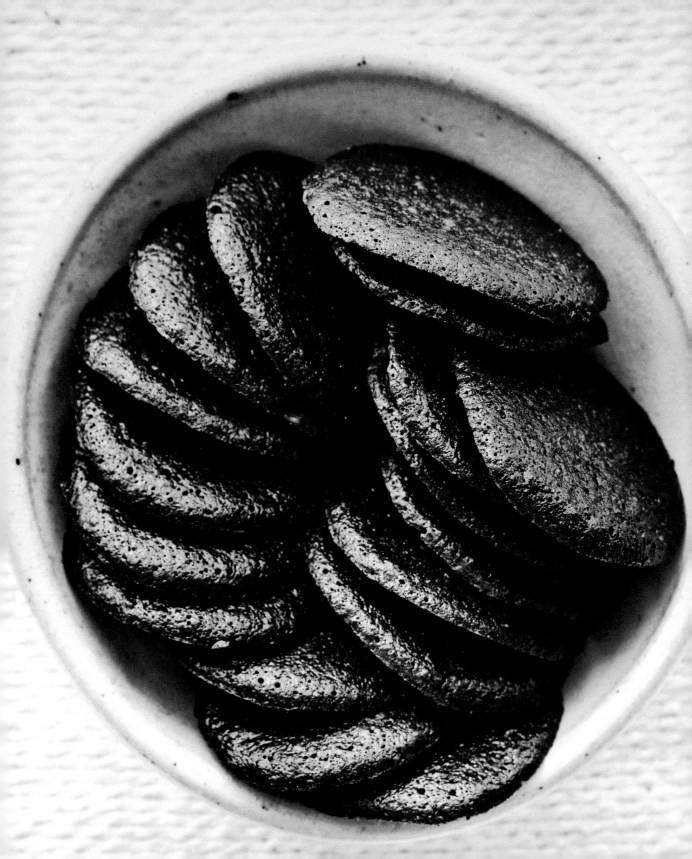

oatmeal crispies

Light and crispy, these delicious oatmeal crisps are a great way to satisfy your sweet tooth with a bit of crunch. With only 9 grams of carbs each, they're the perfect way to jazz up a yogurt bowl, or you can use them as a lower-sugar ice cream topping!

quick & simple | yield: 36 cookies

¾ cup (150 g) coconut sugar

¼ cup (31g) all-purpose flour

¼ tsp baking powder

⅛ tsp salt

½ cup (114 g) unsalted butter, melted

2 large eggs

1 tsp vanilla extract

1 cup (90 g) rolled oats

Preheat your oven to 325°F (163°C) and line two baking sheets with non-stick foil. Set the pans aside.

In a food processor or blender, combine the coconut sugar, flour, baking powder, salt, butter, eggs, vanilla extract, and oats, and process for about a minute, until the oats are ground up.

Drop the batter by ½ tablespoons (8 g), about 2 inches (5 cm) apart, onto the foil-lined baking sheets. Place the pans in the oven, and bake the cookies until they're golden brown and crispy, about 25 minutes.

Remove the pans from the oven. Carefully slide the foil off the baking sheets and let the cookies cool completely. Now, we will carefully peel the cookies off the foil. Make sure to be very light with your touch and gentle when pulling them off the foil . . . they're very delicate cookies!

Store the cookies in a sealed container on the counter for up to 3 days.

Nutrition Info (Serving size: 1 cookie): Calories: 80, Total Fat: 4.5 g, Saturated Fat: 3 g, Total Carbohydrates: 9 g, Sugar: 6 g, Fiber: <1 g, Sodium: 13 mg, Protein: 1 g

high-protein chewy gingersnaps

Ginger is amazing at packing in flavor and adding sweetness without adding additional sugar. These gingersnaps are a perfect chewy texture whether you enjoy them in the morning with a cup of coffee or for an extra bit of protein and sweetness after dinner!

dairy-free | high protein | quick & simple | yield: 12 cookies

1 cup (95 g) almond flour

¼ cup (23 g) rolled oats

¼ tsp baking soda

½ tsp baking powder

½ tbsp (3 g) ground ginger

1 tsp ground cinnamon

1 (15-oz [425-g]) can low-sodium chickpeas, rinsed and drained

¼ cup (65 g) almond butter

1½ tsp (8 ml) vanilla extract

½ cup (120 ml) maple syrup or molasses

Preheat your oven to 350°F (177°C). Line a baking sheet with parchment paper and set it aside.

Next, add the almond flour, oats, baking soda, baking powder, ginger, and cinnamon to the bowl of a large food processor. Process for 15 to 20 seconds, until a uniform powder has formed. Now, add in your chickpeas, almond butter, vanilla extract, and maple syrup. Blend all of the ingredients together for about a minute, until your batter is a smooth consistency. You may need to stop the food processor once or twice and scrape down the sides.

Once the batter is one consistency, remove the blade. Chill the dough for 1 to 2 hours.

Using an ice cream scoop, drop the batter about 2 inches (5 cm) apart onto the prepared baking sheet. With a fork, gently press the dough scoops flat or shape them into your desired cookie shape. (These won't change shape much when you bake them.)

Put your baking sheet in the oven and bake for about 25 minutes, until the cookies are set and have started to brown slightly on the top.

Remove the baking sheet from the oven and let the cookies sit on the pan for about 5 minutes. Then transfer your cookies to a cooling rack.

Store your cookies in an airtight container for up to 3 days or freeze for up to 6 months.

TIPS: For a smoother batter, remove the skins of the chickpeas. Just dry the chickpeas off with a towel after rinsing them and then rub them between two paper towels. Most of the skins will pop right off!

Don't have any almond butter? No worries! You can sub in another nut butter or a cooking oil of your choice.

Nutrition Info (Serving size: 1 cookie): Calories: 151, Total Fat: 7 g, Saturated Fat: <1 g, Total Carbohydrates: 18 g, Sugar: 8 g, Fiber: 3 g, Sodium: 136 mg, Protein: 5 g

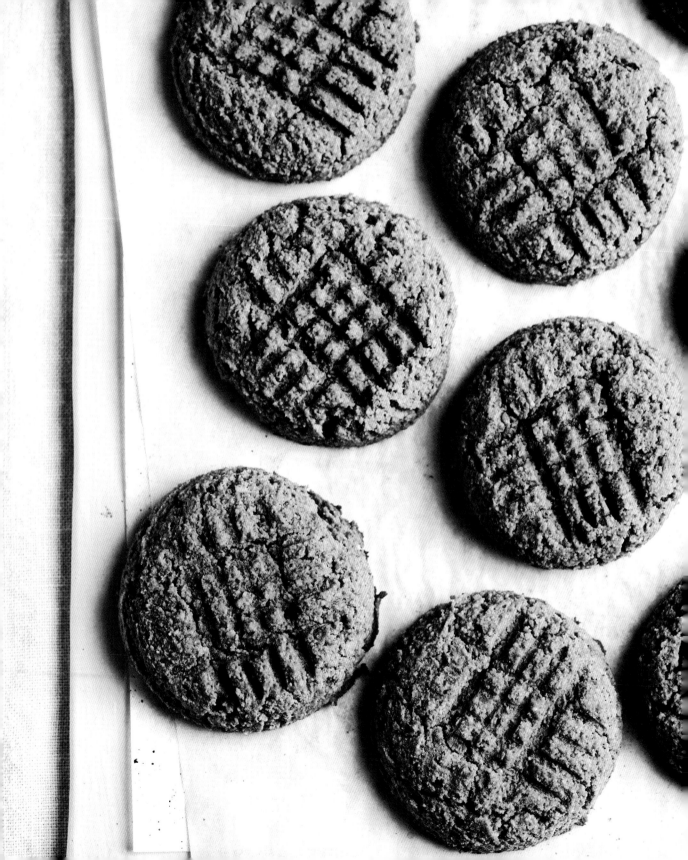

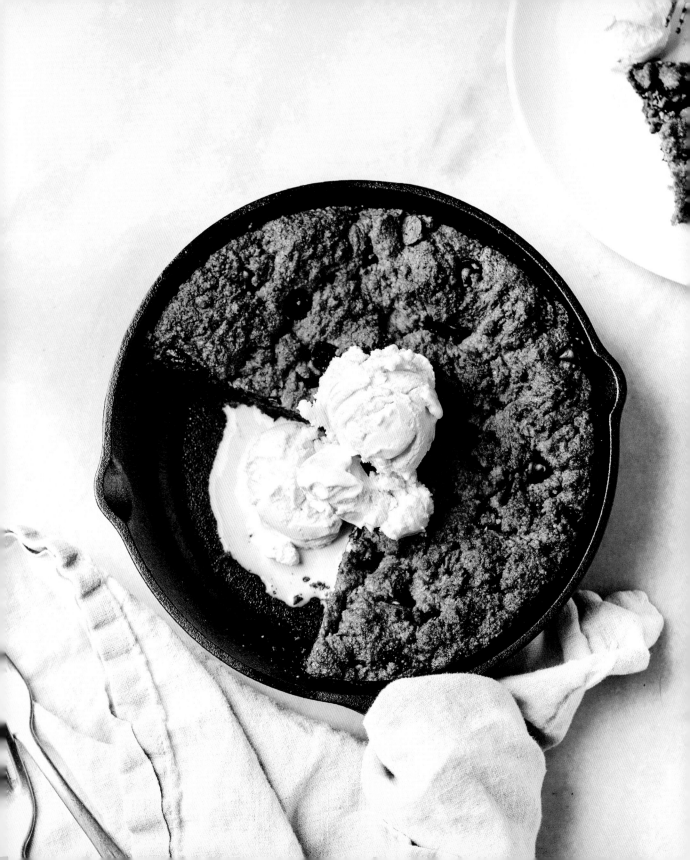

easy chocolate chip skillet cookie

Yes, you read that correctly. A deliciously blood sugar–friendly skillet cookie does exist! The combination of almond flour and tapioca flour in this skillet cookie gives it the perfect fluffy texture, but without a ton of refined carbohydrates. And we're using a bit less sugar than we would in a traditional cookie recipe.

gluten-free | high protein | yield: 12 servings

1⅔ cups (158 g) almond flour

⅓ cup (40 g) tapioca starch/flour

1 tsp baking powder

1 tsp baking soda

½ tsp sea salt

½ cup (100 g) coconut sugar

3 tbsp (45 ml) oil

¼ cup (60 ml) whole milk Greek yogurt

1 large egg, beaten

1 tsp vanilla extract

½ cup (84 g) chocolate chips

Preheat your oven to 350°F (177°C). Spray a properly seasoned cast-iron skillet (or another baking dish of choice) with your favorite cooking oil spray. Set the skillet or pan aside.

In a medium-sized bowl, combine your almond flour, tapioca flour, baking powder, baking soda, salt, and coconut sugar and whisk together until well combined. Set aside.

In a separate bowl, combine your oil, Greek yogurt, egg, and vanilla extract. Whisk them together until well combined. Then, add the oil and milk mixture to the flour mixture and stir them together with a rubber spatula until well combined and a dough has formed. Stir in your chocolate chips.

Spread the dough into your greased skillet or pan. Bake for 25 to 30 minutes, or until a toothpick inserted into the center comes out clean. Remove the skillet or pan from the oven and let it cool for about 20 minutes, until the pan is cool enough to handle safely. Slice and serve!

Store leftovers in an airtight container for up to 2 days, or in the refrigerator for up to 7 days.

TIPS: Try using a no-added-sugar chocolate chip variety to reduce the amount of sugar even more. There are lots of great brands sweetened with stevia, monk fruit, and others.

I know you're going to want to dig in right after this deliciousness comes out of the oven, but try to resist the urge! Those 20 minutes of cooling really help the cookie gel together and not crumble apart.

Nutrition Info (Serving size: 1/12 of skillet): Calories: 200, Total Fat: 12 g, Saturated Fat: 3 g, Total Carbohydrates: 21 g, Sugar: 14 g, Fiber: 2 g, Sodium: 250 mg, Protein: 6 g

pecan praline cookies

These cookies are like eating a slice of pecan pie but in cookie form! With perfectly crisp edges and a chewy center, they're so yummy. And with only 13 grams of carbs, you don't need to worry about huge blood sugar spikes!

gluten-free | yield: 30 cookies

1 cup (109 g) pecan pieces

2 tbsp (28 g) unsalted butter, melted

2 tbsp (25 g) cane sugar

1 tsp ground cinnamon

1 tsp salt, divided

½ cup (114 g) unsalted butter

1 cup packed (220 g) brown sugar

2 large eggs

2 tsp (10 ml) vanilla extract

1 cup (95 g) almond flour

⅔ cup (80 g) tapioca flour

⅓ cup (40 g) coconut flour

1½ tsp (7 g) baking soda

TIP: For crispier cookies, let them cook a bit longer (14 to 15 minutes), or for chewier cookies, go ahead and pull them out of the oven around the 11 to 12 minute mark.

Nutrition Info (Serving size: 1 cookie): Calories: 128, Total Fat: 8 g, Saturated Fat: 3 g, Total Carbohydrates: 13 g, Sugar: 8 g, Fiber: 2 g, Sodium: 150 mg, Protein: 2 g

Before we get to work on making our cookies, we need to make the glazed pecan pieces that we're going to mix into the cookie dough. To start, line a baking sheet with parchment paper and preheat your oven to 400°F (204°C). Then, in a bowl, combine the pecan pieces, 2 tablespoons (28 g) of unsalted butter, sugar, cinnamon, and ½ teaspoon of salt. Toss them all together until well combined. Now, pour the coated pecan pieces onto your parchment-lined pan and bake in your oven for about 10 minutes, until they start to caramelize. Once the pecan pieces are done, remove them from the oven and set the pan aside to allow them to cool.

While the pecan pieces are cooling, we'll mix up our cookie dough. First, lower the temperature on your oven to 350°F (177°C) and line another pan with parchment paper.

Now, to the bowl of a mixer, add the remaining ½ cup (114 g) of butter and the brown sugar and mix them together until fully combined. Then, add in the eggs and vanilla extract and mix again until combined. In a separate bowl, gently whisk the almond flour, tapioca flour, coconut flour, and baking soda together. Then, while the mixer is running, gradually add the flour mixture to the dough until fully combined. Remove the bowl from the mixer and mix in your glazed pecan pieces with a spoon or rubber spatula.

Roll the dough into 1½-inch (4-cm) balls and arrange them on the cookie sheet about 2 inches (5 cm) away from each other. Bake the cookies for 12 to 14 minutes, until they start to turn golden brown and the edges have crisped up.

Remove them from the oven and let them cool for a few minutes before transferring them to a wire rack to cool completely.

Store your cookies in an airtight container on the counter for 2 to 3 days, in the refrigerator for 1 to 2 weeks, or in the freezer for up to 6 months.

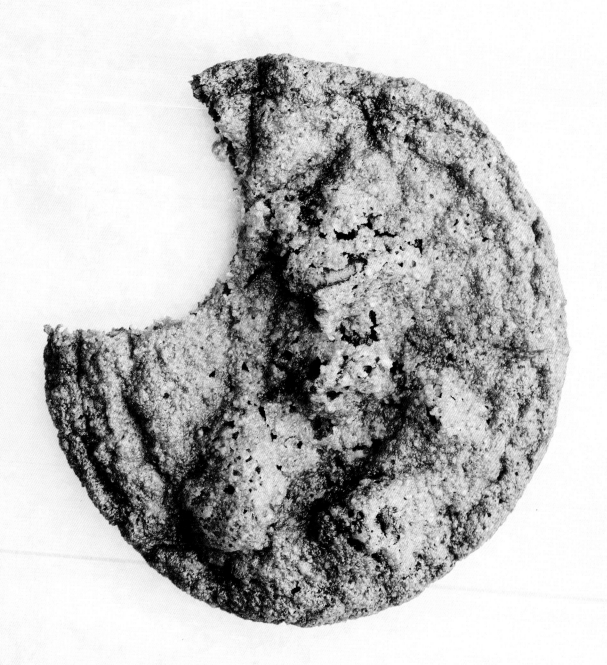

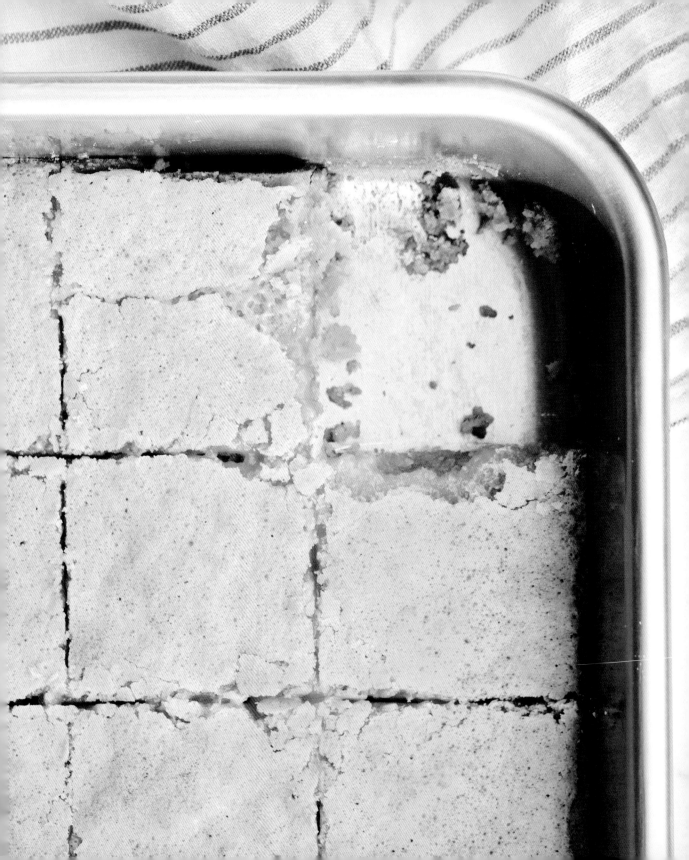

brownies, blondies, & bars . . . oh my!

Get those baking dishes and pans ready, because these bar recipes are going to be some of your new favorites! Oftentimes, people living with diabetes think classic desserts like Nutty Balanced Brownies (page 40) or Grain-Free Lemon Squares (page 44) are off-limits. Whether it's the high saturated fat content or the high sugar content, they definitely seem to be in a category that is reserved for people without diabetes. But again, this is just not true! You absolutely can enjoy these desserts while also living with diabetes. We just need to make a few strategic changes to make them a bit more blood sugar friendly. I'm certain you'll love these diabetes-friendly versions even more than the traditional ones!

Since all of these recipes make quite a few servings/bars, you may want to freeze some of them for another time. And that's definitely doable! I recommend letting all of these recipes cool a bit (if not completely) to room temperature before slicing them. And then, after they've been sliced, arrange them in a single layer in your freezer for a few hours. Then, add them to whatever bag or container you want to store them in long term. Freezing them this way keeps them from sticking together into one big clump, and also makes it super easy to grab one and reheat it whenever you'd like!

nutty balanced brownies

When was the last time you had a deliciously decadent brownie with only 6 grams of sugar? Never? Well, we're about change that! These brownies are deliciously fluffy and perfectly blood sugar friendly. And my favorite part is just how perfectly they satisfy any sweet tooth!

quick & simple | yield: 16 brownies

⅓ cup (80 ml) unsweetened applesauce

2 tbsp (30 ml) maple syrup

⅓ cup (76 g) unsalted butter, melted

1 large egg, beaten

1 tsp vanilla extract

1 cup (95 g) almond flour

½ cup (45 g) rolled oats

¼ cup (22 g) unsweetened cocoa powder

½ tsp baking soda

½ tsp baking powder

½ cup (84 g) chocolate chips or chocolate chunks, divided

2 tbsp (14 g) chopped pecans

2 tbsp (14 g) chopped walnuts

Preheat your oven to 375°F (191°C) and grease a 9 x 9–inch (23 x 23–cm) pan with your preferred cooking oil spray. (You can also line it with parchment paper if you'd prefer.) Set it aside.

Now, in a large bowl, combine the applesauce, maple syrup, melted butter, egg, and vanilla extract. Whisk them together well until they form a uniform mixture. Then set that bowl aside.

Now, in a blender or food processor, add the almond flour, oats, cocoa powder, baking soda, and baking powder and process until everything is combined and the oats are ground up, 15 to 20 seconds. Add this dry mixture to the wet ingredients mixed together previously and stir it with a whisk until fully combined. (The batter may be a bit lumpy, but that's okay!) Then, mix in ¼ cup (42 g) of the chocolate chips.

Pour the batter into the prepared pan. Sprinkle the chopped pecans and chopped walnuts on top of the batter along with the remaining ¼ cup (42 g) of chocolate chips. Place the pan in the oven and bake for 20 minutes, or until a knife or toothpick inserted in the center comes out clean. Let the brownies cool for a bit before slicing into them.

Store cut brownies in an airtight container on the counter for up to 3 days, in the refrigerator for up to 7 days, or in the freezer for up to 6 months.

TIP: Feel free to swap out the nuts for different toppings to mix up the flavors a bit!

Nutrition Info (Serving size: 1 brownie): Calories: 144, Total Fat: 11 g, Saturated Fat: 4 g, Total Carbohydrates: 12 g, Sugar: 6 g, Fiber: 2 g, Sodium: 45 mg, Protein: 3.5 g

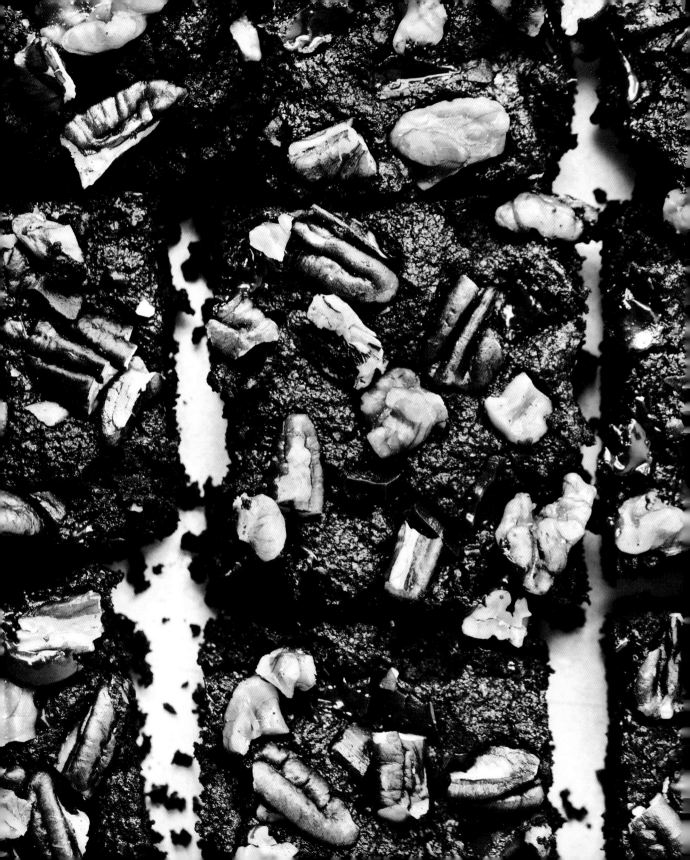

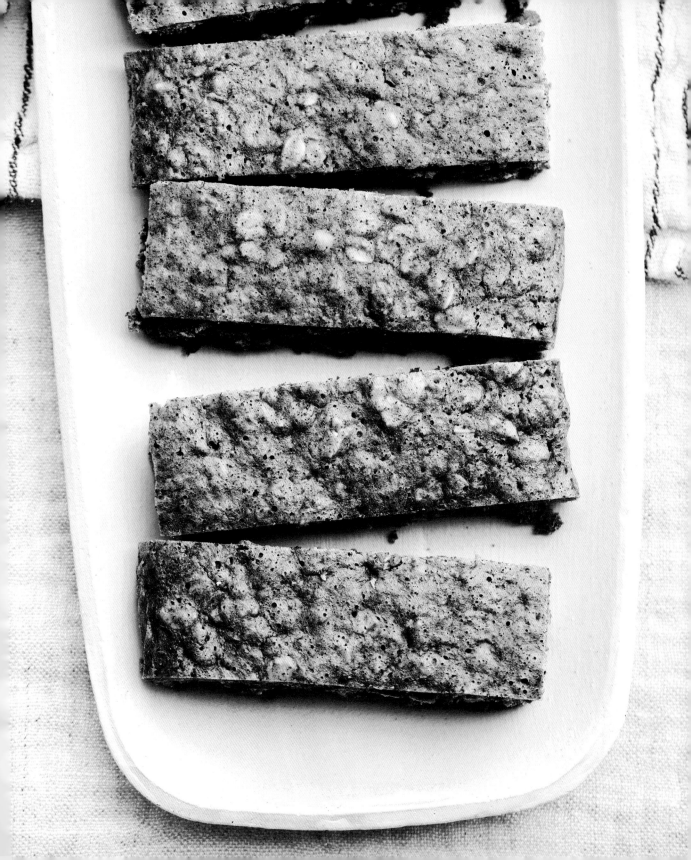

banana cashew blondies

These banana bread–inspired blondies are fluffy and decadent at the same time. Traditional blondies come loaded with sugar and not much else, but not these blondies! They pack in 5 grams of protein into each bar, which not only makes them more satisfying but also helps promote more stable blood sugars after you enjoy one.

dairy-free | high protein | quick & simple | yield: 12 bars

½ cup (129 g) cashew butter

¼ cup (60 ml) maple syrup

2 large (or 3 small) ripe bananas, mashed

2 large eggs, beaten

1 tsp vanilla extract

½ tsp almond extract

1¼ cups (113 g) rolled oats, ground

¼ cup (30 g) tapioca flour

½ tsp baking soda

½ tsp cinnamon

To start, preheat your oven to 350°F (177°C) and grease a 9 x 9–inch (23 x 23–cm) square baking pan. (You can also line it with parchment paper if you prefer.) Set the pan aside.

In a medium-sized bowl, combine the cashew butter, maple syrup, mashed bananas, eggs, and extracts. Thoroughly whisk them all together until they are one uniform consistency. Set this bowl aside. Now, in a second medium-sized bowl, combine your ground oats, tapioca flour, baking soda, and cinnamon and whisk them together real quick to combine them a bit. Add the dry mixture to your wet ingredients and stir it all together using a rubber spatula until just combined and there is no more dry flour in the bowl.

Pour the batter into your prepared baking pan, and place the pan in the oven. Bake for 20 to 25 minutes, until a toothpick inserted in the center comes out clean and the top has started to turn golden brown.

Remove the pan from the oven and let your blondies cool for 10 to 15 minutes before trying to cut into them.

Store your cut blondies in an airtight container on the counter for up to 5 days. I recommend placing a paper towel inside whatever container you use to help absorb any moisture and prevent mold from forming. You can also freeze your blondies for up to 6 months in a sealed container.

TIP: Not into cashews? No problem . . . any unsweetened nut butter will work in this recipe!

Nutrition Info (Serving size: 1 bar): Calories: 162, Total Fat: 7 g, Saturated Fat: 1.5 g, Total Carbohydrates: 22 g, Sugar: 7 g, Fiber: 2 g, Sodium: 67 mg, Protein: 5 g

grain-free lemon squares

It doesn't get more classic than a warm, chewy lemon square. Except my grain-free version offers a more blood sugar–friendly crust, and we've cut way back on the sugar in the filling . . . but I promise you'll be so blown away by how delicious they are, you'll never notice, or realize, that they also pack 5 grams of protein per square!

gluten-free | high protein | yield: 16 bars

CRUST

2 cups (190 g) almond flour

¼ cup (50 g) granulated sugar

4 tbsp (57 g) butter, room temperature

1 large egg

½ tbsp (3 g) lemon zest

FILLING

2 large eggs

1 cup (200 g) granulated sugar

3 tbsp (23 g) tapioca starch

½ tsp baking powder

½ tbsp (3 g) lemon zest

3 tbsp (45 ml) lemon juice

1 tsp vanilla extract

Preheat your oven to 350°F (177°C) and grease a 9 x 9–inch (23 x 23–cm) baking dish well with butter or cooking spray. Set the dish aside.

Now, to the bowl of a large food processor, add all of your crust ingredients. Using the S-blade attachment, process the ingredients until a dough ball has formed, about 10 seconds. Then, carefully transfer the mixture to your greased baking dish. Press the mixture down into the bottom of the dish. Bake the crust for 10 to 11 minutes, just until it starts to turn golden brown. Remove the crust from the oven and set it aside.

To make the filling, in a separate bowl, combine the eggs and the sugar and whisk thoroughly for 30 to 45 seconds. Next, add in the tapioca starch and baking powder and whisk again for 15 to 20 seconds. Finally, add the lemon zest, lemon juice, and vanilla extract and whisk until combined. Pour the filling over your crust. (Make sure the crust has cooled a bit; we don't want scrambled eggs in our lemon bars!)

Place the pan in the oven and bake for 20 to 25 minutes, until set and the top is slightly brown. Remove the bars from the oven and let them cool completely. Cut and enjoy!

Store your lemon bars in an airtight container in the refrigerator for up to 1 week.

TIP: Normally, I would use something other than granulated sugar in a recipe like this, but there's something about getting that classic yellow color of lemon squares that is so appealing! But, if you're ok with the color changing some, feel free to use any other granulated sweetener in the filling.

Nutrition Info (Serving size: 1 bar): Calories: 181, Total Fat: 9 g, Saturated Fat: 3 g, Total Carbohydrates: 20 g, Sugar: 16 g, Fiber: 2 g, Sodium: 14 mg, Protein: 5 g

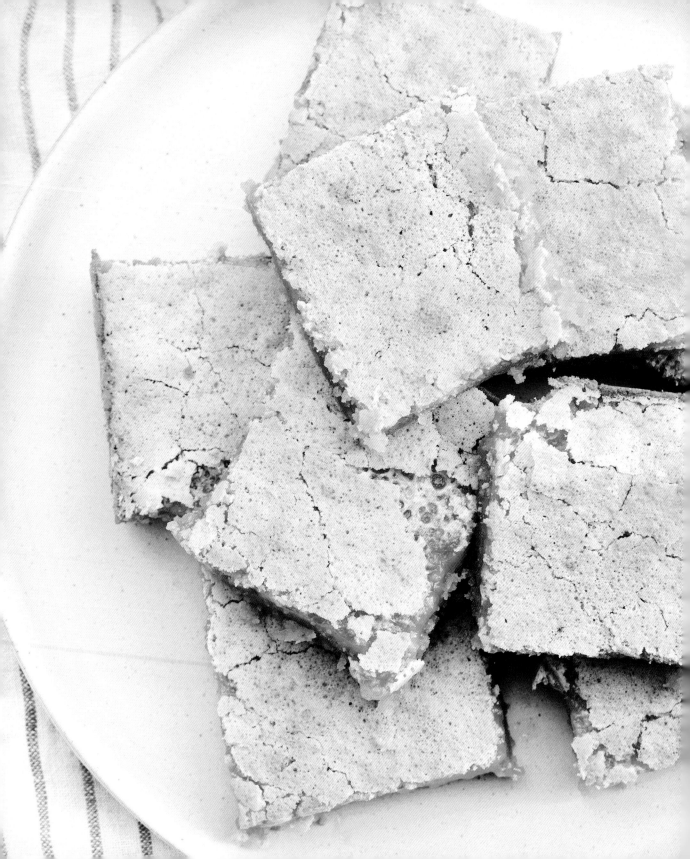

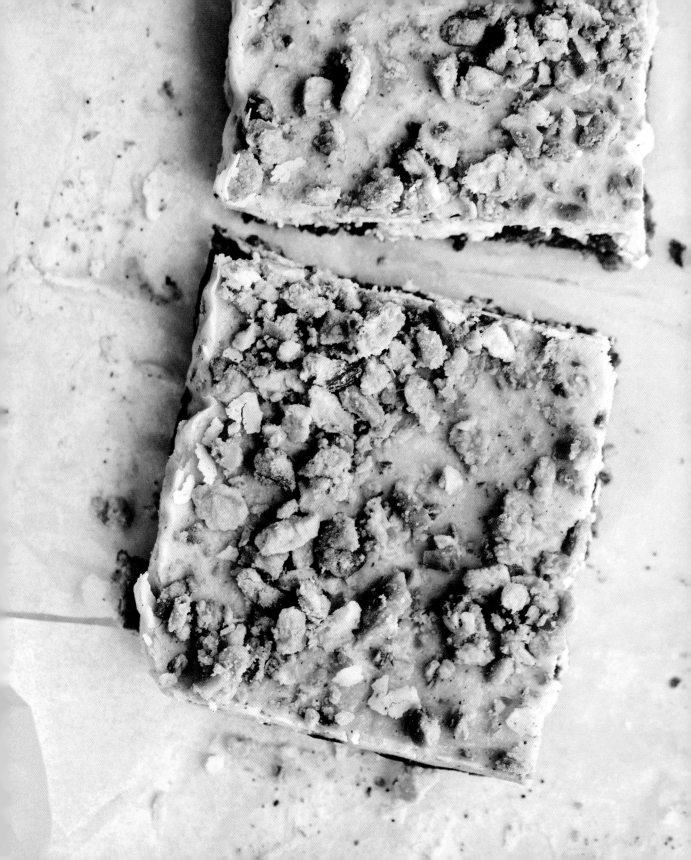

apple pie cheesecake bars

This recipe tastes like a warm slice of apple pie . . . except it's cold and you don't have to bake it! These Apple Pie Cheesecake Bars require zero cooking and have the smoothest, creamiest texture! They're perfect for a blood sugar–balancing treat after dinner or just because.

gluten-free | yield: 12 bars

CRUST

⅓ cup (48 g) raw almonds

6 Medjool dates (120 g), pitted

2 tbsp (5 g) crushed apple chips or dehydrated apples

½ tsp almond extract

¼ tsp salt

1 tsp cinnamon

FILLING

8 oz (224 g) cream cheese, softened

½ cup (120 ml) plain nonfat Greek yogurt

1 tbsp (14 g) brown sugar, packed

2 oz (60 ml) apple juice

2 tbsp (27 g) coconut oil

½ tsp cinnamon

½ tsp nutmeg

2 tbsp (5 g) crushed apple chips or dehydrated apples

First, line an 8 x 8–inch (20 x 20–cm) or 9 x 9–inch (23 x 23–cm) square pan with parchment paper or foil and set it aside.

For the crust, in the bowl of a large food processor, combine the almonds, dates, apple chips, almond extract, salt, and cinnamon. Pulse until the mixture resembles large grains of sand and is slightly sticky. This should take about 30 seconds.

Add the crust mixture to your parchment-lined pan. Then, firmly press the crust down into the bottom of the pan.

For the filling, you're going to need to give your food processor a quick rinse. Then, add the cream cheese, Greek yogurt, brown sugar, apple juice, coconut oil, cinnamon, and nutmeg to the clean bowl of the food processor and process until smooth. Pour the filling on top of the crust. Sprinkle the remaining crushed apple chips on top.

Set the pan in the refrigerator for 3 to 4 hours so it can firm up. Once firm, slice and enjoy!

These Apple Pie Cheesecake Bars will keep for up to 7 days in the fridge or up to 3 months in the freezer.

> TIP: Look for apple chips in the bulk section of your local grocery store or in the dried fruit section.

Nutrition Info (Serving size: 1 bar): Calories: 162, Total Fat: 11 g, Saturated Fat: 6 g, Total Carbohydrates: 14 g, Sugar: 11 g, Fiber: 2 g, Sodium: 124 mg, Protein: 3 g

brownie batter energy bars

I decided to call these Brownie Batter Energy Bars because they're equal parts decadent and energizing. They also offer a quality source of protein to help promote stable blood sugars throughout your day.

high protein | quick & simple | yield: 12 bars

1½ cups (135 g) rolled oats

½ cup (44 g) unsweetened cocoa powder

⅓ cup (80 ml) maple syrup

¼ cup (65 g) unsweetened almond butter

1 large egg

½ cup (120 ml) plain low-fat Greek yogurt

1 tsp vanilla extract

1 tsp almond extract

½ cup (84 g) chocolate chips or other mix-ins

Preheat your oven to 350°F (177°C). Then, line a 9 x 9–inch (23 x 23–cm) baking pan with parchment paper and set it aside. (You can also use one of those cool silicone bar-shaped pans if you have one!)

Now, in a medium-sized bowl, add your oats and cocoa powder and whisk to combine. Then, in a separate bowl, add the maple syrup, almond butter, egg, Greek yogurt, vanilla extract, and almond extract. Whisk thoroughly until combined. Then add this mixture to the bowl with the oats and cocoa powder. Mix your batter together until fully combined. Add your chocolate chips to the bowl and stir until combined.

Pour the batter into your pan and spread it out evenly. Place the pan in the oven and bake for 25 to 30 minutes, until a toothpick inserted in the center comes out clean. Let the bars cool for 15 to 20 minutes before slicing them.

Store cut bars on the counter for up to 5 days or in the freezer for up to 6 months.

TIP: If you prefer the classic chocolate peanut butter combo over just plain chocolate, feel free to use peanut butter instead of almond butter!

Nutrition Info (Serving size: 1 bar): Calories: 173, Total Fat: 8 g, Saturated Fat: 3 g, Total Carbohydrates: 24 g, Sugar: 11 g, Fiber: 3 g, Sodium: 11 mg, Protein: 5 g

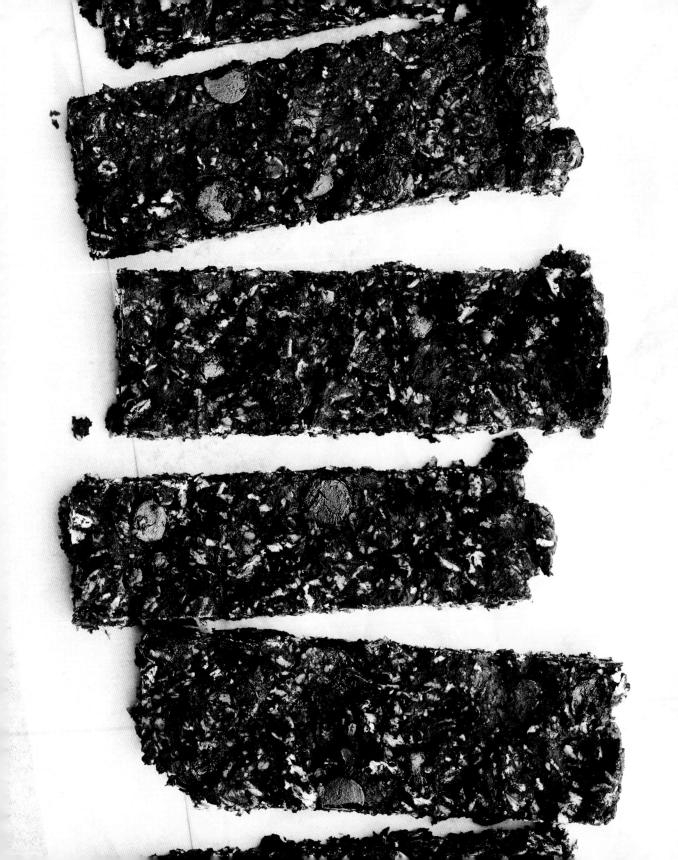

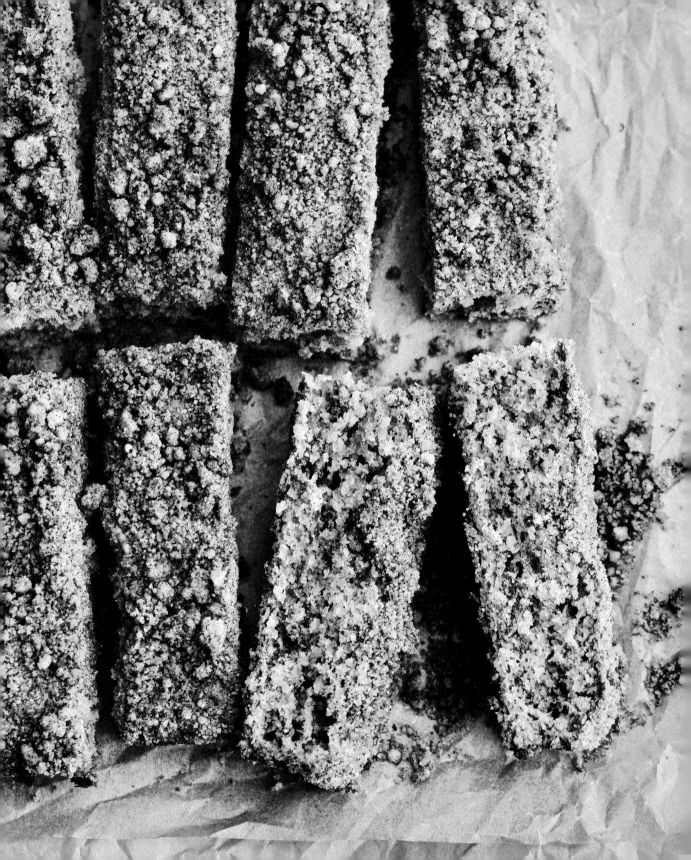

cinnamon coffee cake bars

Traditional coffee cakes are typically loaded with sugar and will send blood sugars spiking, only to be followed by a crash later on. But not my coffee cake bars! These bars use nutrient-dense ingredients like oats and Greek yogurt for the cake layer, and a lot less sugar. And thanks to the delicious streusel layer, they still taste amazing!

quick & simple | yield: 12 bars

1 cup (90 g) rolled oats

¼ cup (30 g) tapioca flour

½ tsp baking soda

1 tsp baking powder

½ tsp salt

4 tbsp (57 g) unsalted butter, softened

¾ cup (150 g) granulated sugar, divided

1 large egg

½ cup (120 ml) plain low-fat Greek yogurt

1 tsp vanilla extract

¼ cup (31 g) all-purpose flour

2 tsp (5 g) cinnamon

2 tbsp (28 g) unsalted butter, melted

Preheat your oven to 350°F (177°C) and grease an 8 x 8–inch (20 x 20–cm) or 9 x 9–inch (23 x 23–cm) baking pan. Set it aside.

Add your oats to a food processor or blender and grind them up until a powder forms. Add the ground oats, tapioca flour, baking soda, baking powder, and salt to a bowl and stir to combine.

Next, add the 4 tablespoons (57 g) of softened butter, ½ cup (100 g) of sugar, egg, Greek yogurt, and vanilla extract to another bowl and whisk together until fully combined. Add this mixture to the ground oat mixture and stir until just combined with a rubber spatula.

Add half of the batter to the prepared baking pan. Now, in another bowl, we're going to mix up our streusel topping. Simply combine the flour, ¼ cup (50 g) of granulated sugar, cinnamon, and melted butter in a bowl and mix to combine. The streusel will clump up and resemble wet sand. Sprinkle half of it evenly over the coffee cake batter. Then add the second half of the batter on top of that, and then finally sprinkle the second half of the streusel on top of that.

Place your pan in the oven and bake for 25 to 30 minutes, or until the top of the coffee cake bars start to turn golden brown and a toothpick inserted in the center comes out clean. Remove the pan from the oven and let the bars cool for 15 to 20 minutes before slicing.

Store cut bars on the counter for up to 5 days or in the freezer for up to 6 months.

Nutrition Info (Serving size: 1 bar): Calories: 157, Total Fat: 7 g, Saturated Fat: 4 g, Total Carbohydrates: 22 g, Sugar: 13 g, Fiber: 1 g, Sodium: 160 mg, Protein: 3 g

TIP: If you enjoy the flavor of just the cake by itself, feel free to leave the streusel topping off!

low-carb magic bars

Imagine the classic coconut and chocolate-infused magic bars we love, but made nutrient rich and blood sugar friendly! These magic bars are made with almond flour and almond butter for a lower-carb alternative, and we pile on nutrient-dense toppings like hemp seeds, pecans, and coconut. The end result is a deliciously classic blood sugar–friendly treat!

dairy-free | gluten-free | high protein | quick & simple | yield: 12 bars

1 ½ cups (143 g) almond flour

1 tsp cinnamon

½ tsp baking powder

¼ tsp sea salt

½ cup (130 g) unsweetened almond butter

⅓ cup (80 ml) pure maple syrup

1 large egg, beaten

1 tbsp (6 g) unsweetened coconut flakes

1 tbsp (10 g) hemp seeds

2 tbsp (21 g) dark chocolate chunks or chips

2 tbsp (14 g) pecan pieces

Preheat your oven to 350°F (177°C). Line or grease a loaf pan and set aside.

In a medium-sized mixing bowl, combine the almond flour, cinnamon, baking powder, and sea salt. Whisk them together to combine well. Add in the almond butter, maple syrup, and egg, and mix it all together using a rubber spatula. It will be crumbly and slightly dry looking. Press the dough down into the prepared loaf pan.

Now, in a small bowl, mix the unsweetened coconut flakes, hemp seeds, dark chocolate chunks, and pecan pieces. Spread them evenly over the top of the dough in the loaf pan.

Place the pan in the oven and bake the bars for 20 to 25 minutes, until the edges spring back to the touch.

Remove the bars from the oven and let them cool completely in the pan. Once cooled, you can slice into the bars and enjoy!

Store these bars in the refrigerator in an airtight container for up to 7 days.

TIPS: You can switch up the toppings for different flavor combinations! (Just remember, that could change the nutritional information, so make sure to adjust any medication doses as needed/indicated.)

Don't try to cut the bars before they have had a chance to cool! They may fall apart on you if you try.

Nutrition Info (Serving size: 1 bar): Calories: 196, Total Fat: 14 g, Saturated Fat: 2 g, Total Carbohydrates: 13 g, Sugar: 7 g, Fiber: 3 g, Sodium: 57 mg, Protein: 6 g

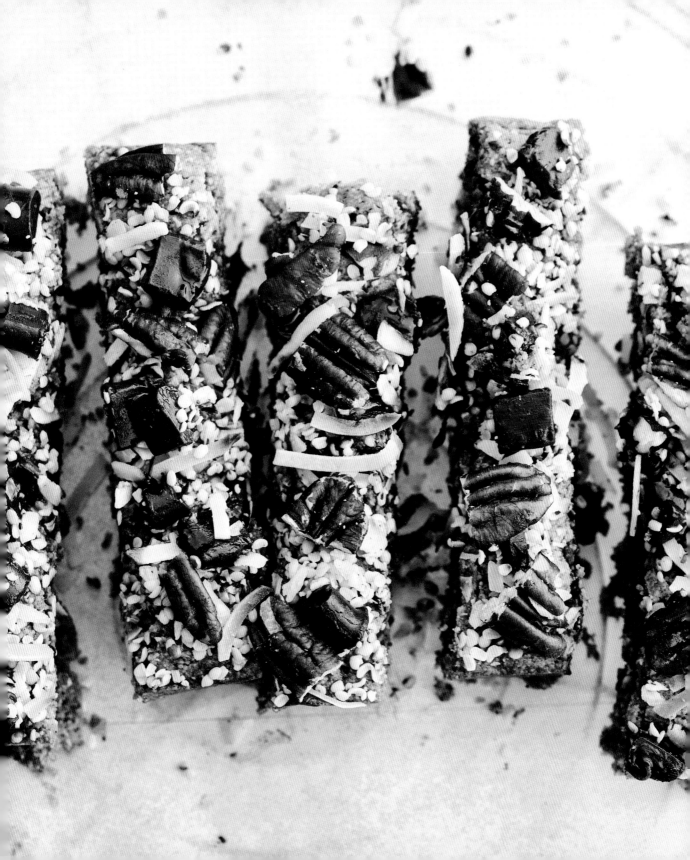

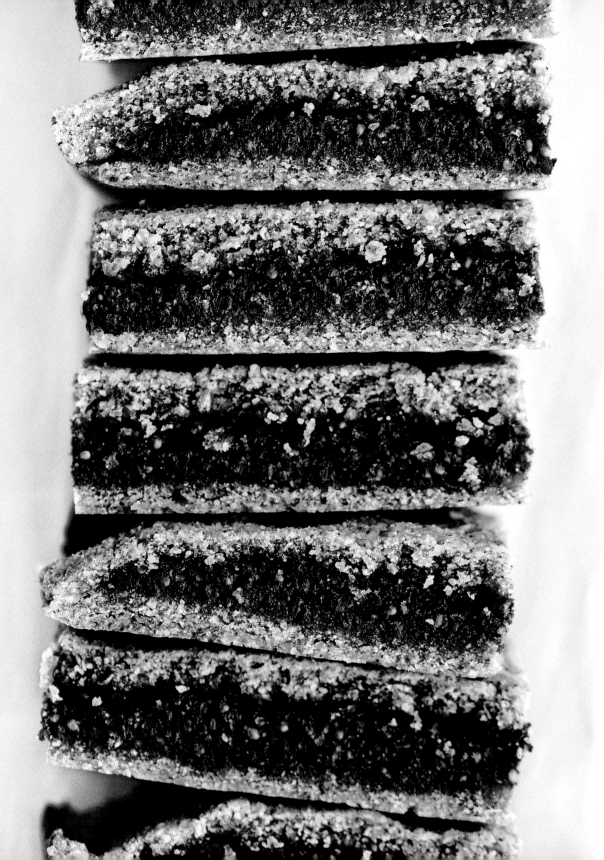

grain-free fig bars

These bars are a more balanced version of that classic Fig Newton–style bar we all loved as kids. With 3 grams of fiber, 2 grams of protein, and a low amount of added sugar, they'll satisfy that sweet tooth without sending blood sugars sky high.

dairy-free | gluten-free | yield: 16 bars

¾ cup (71 g) almond flour

¼ cup (30 g) coconut flour

½ cup (60 g) tapioca flour or arrowroot powder

2 tsp (5 g) cinnamon

¼ cup (61 g) pumpkin puree

¼ cup (60 ml) unsweetened applesauce

2 tbsp (30 ml) maple syrup

5 oz (140 g) dried figs

TIP: This dough is sticky! As mentioned above, it's really important to use wet hands when handling it! And if you want to try different types of fruit filling, you can use other dried fruits like raisins, blueberries, or mangoes— just remember to adjust the nutritional information accordingly.

Preheat your oven to 350°F (177°C) and line an 8 x 8–inch (20 x 20–cm) pan with parchment paper. Set the pan aside.

In a bowl, combine the almond flour, coconut flour, tapioca flour, and cinnamon and mix to combine. Then, add in the pumpkin puree, apple-sauce, and maple syrup. Mix thoroughly until a dough forms. Press half the mixture into the bottom of your pan. (The dough will be sticky. It helps to wet your fingertips slightly with cold water before handling the dough, or chill the dough for an hour before handling it.)

Next, in a small saucepan, boil the figs with just enough water to cover them for 5 to 10 minutes. Remove the figs from the heat and drain the water. Add the figs to a food processor and process until smooth, about 30 seconds. Spread the fig mixture over the crust in the loaf pan, leaving a small edge all the way around each side.

Next, you're going to add the second half of the dough on top of the fig mixture. Using wet fingers and hands, add small flat pieces of dough on top until the entire pan is covered again (almost like you're piecing them all together). Gently press the dough edges together to seal the fig mixture inside.

Bake the bars for 25 minutes, or until the top is golden brown. Immediately after removing the pan from the oven, lift the fig bars out of the pan using the parchment paper and place them on a wire rack to cool. Carefully, using a wide/flat spatula, slide the parchment paper out from under the bars. Let the bars cool completely on the wire rack before slicing.

Store cut bars in the refrigerator for up to 5 days, or in the freezer for up to 6 months.

Nutrition Info (Serving size: 1 bar): Calories: 78, Total Fat: 2 g, Saturated Fat: <1 g, Total Carbohydrates: 14 g, Sugar: 7 g, Fiber: 3 g, Sodium: 4 mg, Protein: 2 g

fluffy monster cookie bars

My Fluffy Monster Cookie Bars capture that classic flavor combo of oatmeal, peanut butter, and chocolate, but without a ton of extra sugar! These bars are perfect for a satisfying after-dinner treat or a filling midday snack!

high protein | quick & simple | yield: 16 bars

1 cup (258 g) creamy unsweetened peanut butter

¼ cup (57 g) unsalted butter, softened

2 tbsp (25 g) granulated sugar

¼ cup (55 g) brown sugar, packed

2 large eggs

1 tsp vanilla extract

2 cups (180 g) rolled oats

¾ cup (71 g) almond flour

½ tsp baking soda

1 tsp baking powder

¼ cup (42 g) chocolate chips

1 oz (28 g) chocolate morsel candies (like M&Ms®)

Preheat your oven to 375°F (191°C). Grease an 8 x 8–inch (20 x 20–cm) or 9 x 9–inch (23 x 23–cm) square pan and set it aside.

Now, in the bowl of a stand mixer, combine the peanut butter, butter, granulated sugar, and brown sugar and beat on medium speed for 2 to 3 minutes, until well combined. Next, add in the eggs and vanilla extract and beat for about 30 more seconds.

In a separate bowl, combine the oats, almond flour, baking soda, and baking powder and whisk gently to combine. Add this dry mixture to the wet mixture in the stand mixer bowl. Mix on medium speed for 1 to 2 minutes, until a dough has formed. Remove the bowl from the mixer and mix the chocolate chips in by hand.

Spread the dough into your greased pan. Top the dough with the chocolate candies and gently press them down. Bake the bars for about 20 minutes, or until a toothpick inserted in the center comes out clean. Let the pan cool for 20 to 25 minutes before cutting into your bars.

Store the bars on the counter in an airtight container for up to 5 days or in the freezer for up to 3 months.

TIPS: If you want to mix up the flavor a bit, feel free to use a different type of nut butter!

Some of my favorite unsweetened peanut butter brands are actually in-house store brands! Stores like Costco, Whole Foods, Kroger, and more have several options.

Nutrition Info (Serving size: 1 bar): Calories: 240, Total Fat: 16 g, Saturated Fat: 5 g, Total Carbohydrates: 20 g, Sugar: 10 g, Fiber: 3 g, Sodium: 77 mg, Protein: 8 g

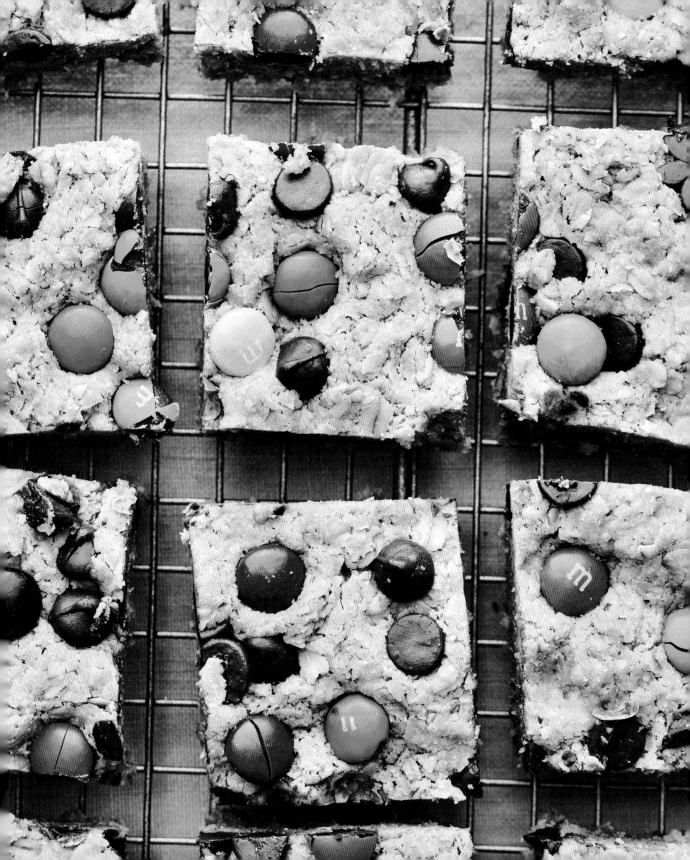

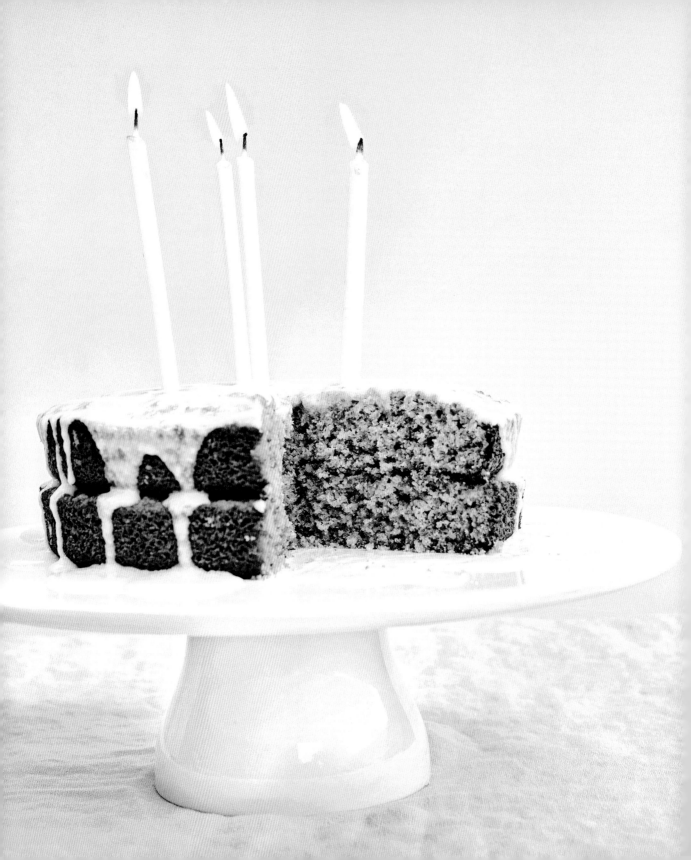

let's celebrate with cakes & pies

Special occasions like birthdays and holidays can be one of the most difficult times to navigate this dilemma of diabetes and dessert. And while one sugar-laden dessert isn't going to completely undo any health journey or blood sugar–management progress you've been on, it is a tough choice when you're the one with diabetes. It feels like every time you're faced with the option of just enjoying the "real thing" but feeling sick afterwards (because of high blood sugars) . . . or being forced to have some diet dessert that tastes like sweetened cardboard.

The recipes in this chapter are the perfect solution to this dilemma! From Funfetti Birthday Cake (page 66) to holiday classics like my Classic Pumpkin Pie (page 70) and Maple Pecan Pie with Almond Flour Crust (page 79), we've taken those classic special occasion desserts and made them blood sugar friendly and delicious. We can use a higher-protein, lower-carbohydrate flour in cakes, or even less sugar in a pie filling, and get an equally delicious dessert! So, you can quite literally have your cake and eat it too!

As you look through the recipes, you'll notice we use similar recipes for the crusts in each of the pies. And we did the same thing with the cake recipes. Once you find a good base recipe that you know works, it's the perfect canvas for adding in the flavorings and mix-ins you want!

chocolate cheesecake with hazelnut-spiced crust

Cheesecake was one of the first desserts I ever learned to make in a way that was good for blood sugars! The fat and protein content of cream cheese and plain yogurt actually lend themselves to a nice blood sugar–friendly dessert. And the flavors are so rich, you'll never notice we cut back on some of the sugar.

gluten-free | high protein | yield: 16 slices

CRUST

2 cups (180 g) almond flour

½ cup (58 g) chopped hazelnuts

½ tsp cinnamon

6 tbsp (84 g) unsalted butter, melted

½ cup (100 g) coconut sugar

FILLING

3 (8-oz [224-g]) packages low-fat cream cheese, room temperature

1 cup (200 g) coconut sugar

⅓ cup (29 g) unsweetened cocoa powder

½ tsp ground cinnamon

¼ tsp ground nutmeg

3 large eggs, room temperature

1½ cups (360 ml) plain low-fat yogurt, room temperature

1 tsp vanilla extract

½ tsp almond extract

Preheat your oven to 325°F (163°C). Now, wrap the outside (bottom and sides) of a round springform pan in several layers of foil.

For the crust, to the bowl of your food processor, add your almond flour, hazelnuts, ½ teaspoon of cinnamon, melted butter, and ½ cup (100 g) of coconut sugar. Mix/pulse until the mixture resembles wet sand. Then, press the crust mixture into your foil-wrapped pan. You can press the crust mixture on the bottom only or up the sides too. Then, set the pan aside.

To make the filling, using the whisk attachment of a stand or hand mixer, beat your cream cheese, 1 cup (200 g) of coconut sugar, cocoa powder, ½ teaspoon of cinnamon, and nutmeg until fluffy. Add in your eggs one at a time and beat. Then, add in your yogurt, vanilla extract, and almond extract. Finally, pour the batter into the pan with your crust.

Now, we need to prep a water bath for the cheesecake before baking it. Using a water bath ensures the sides of the cheesecake don't get too hot or overcook.

Place your foil-wrapped springform pan inside of a large rectangle-shaped pan. Add water to the larger pan until it is about halfway up the side of your springform pan.

(continued)

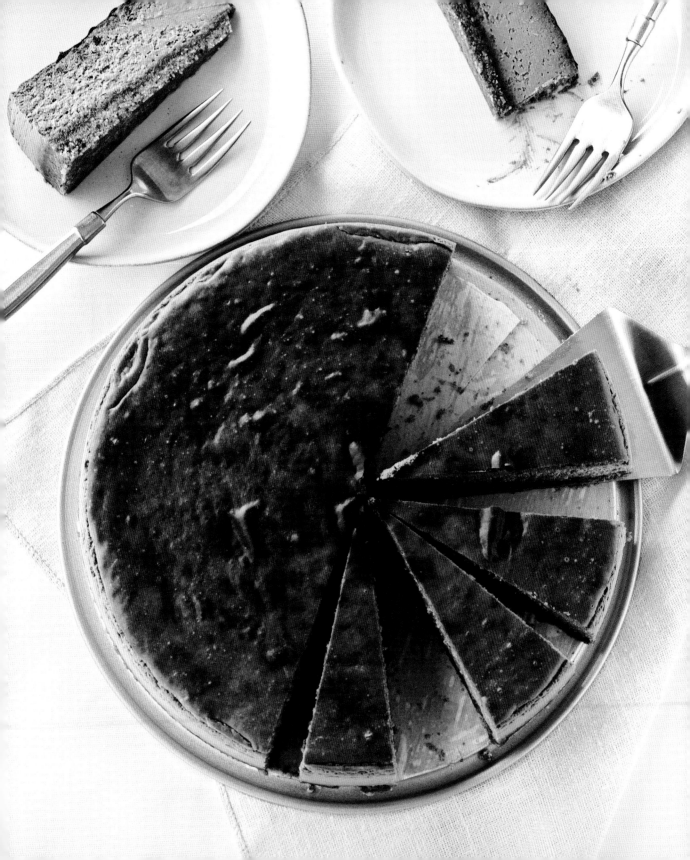

chocolate cheesecake with hazelnut-spiced crust (cont.)

Place the cheesecake (in the water bath) into the oven and bake for 90 minutes, or until the center is set, but it still jiggles slightly. Remove the pan from the oven and carefully pull the cheesecake pan out of the water bath. Let it cool to room temperature. Once cooled, place the cheesecake in the refrigerator or freezer.

Store the cheesecake (covered) in the refrigerator for up to 1 week and in the freezer for up to 1 month.

TIP: A springform pan allows you to remove the sides of the pan, so you can easily cut and serve a beautiful piece of cheesecake. If you don't have a springform pan, you can use a standard 8- or 9-inch (20- or 23-cm) cake pan, but keep in mind, it will take a little bit more finessing to get the cheesecake out of the pan. Or, if you're wondering what pan to place the springform pan inside of and fill with water, a large roasting pan works great!

Nutrition Info (Serving size: 1 slice): Calories: 330, Total Fat: 22 g, Saturated Fat: 9 g, Total Carbohydrates: 27 g, Sugar: 23 g, Fiber: 3 g, Sodium: 222 mg, Protein: 10 g

chocolate coconut cream pie

Get ready, because this Chocolate Coconut Cream Pie is going to blow your socks off!
It's rich and decadent, but with approximately 20 grams of carbohydrates and 7 grams of
protein in each slice, it won't leave your blood sugars skyrocketing. This is the perfect blood
sugar–friendly special occasion pie!

high protein | yield: 16 slices

CRUST

2 cups (180 g) almond flour

½ cup (45 g) rolled oats

¼ cup (50 g) coconut sugar

4 tbsp (57 g) unsalted butter

1 large egg

½ tsp vanilla extract

½ tsp almond extract

FILLING

¼ cup (30 g) coconut flour

¼ cup (22 g) unsweetened
cocoa powder

6 oz (168 g) low-fat cream cheese

⅔ cup (160 ml) plain low-fat
Greek yogurt

⅔ cup (160 ml) maple syrup

1 tsp vanilla extract

First, we're going to prepare our crust. Preheat your oven to 350°F
(177°C) and grease a 9-inch (23-cm) pie plate (or a deep dish
8-inch [20-cm] pie plate) well with butter or cooking spray. Set the
pie plate aside.

Now, to the bowl of a large food processor, add the almond flour, oats,
coconut sugar, butter, egg, vanilla extract, and almond extract. Using
the S-blade attachment, process the ingredients until a dough ball has
formed, about 10 seconds. Then, carefully transfer the mixture to your
greased pie plate. Press the mixture down into the bottom of the pan
and all the way up the sides. Bake the pie crust for 13 to 14 minutes,
until it starts to turn golden brown.

While the crust is baking, we can get our filling ready. You'll need to
use your food processor again, so give the bowl and blade a quick
wash before starting the filling. Once you've done that, add the coconut
flour, cocoa powder, cream cheese, Greek yogurt, maple syrup, and
vanilla extract to the clean bowl of the food processor. Process the filling
for about 20 seconds, until smooth.

Once the pie crust has cooled, carefully add the filling to the pie plate
and spread it out evenly.

(continued)

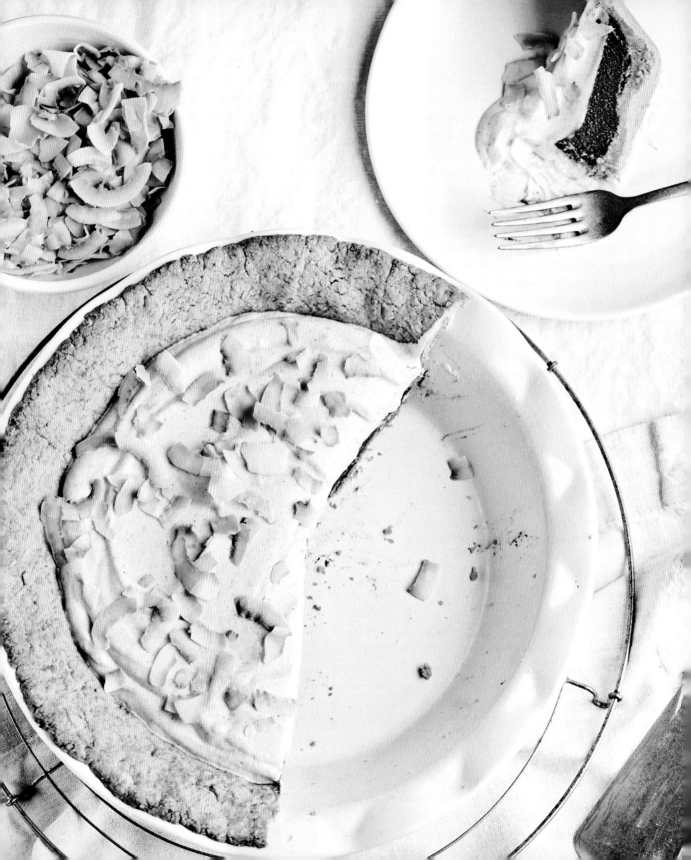

chocolate coconut cream pie (cont.)

COCONUT WHIPPED TOPPING

1 (13.5-oz [400-ml]) can coconut cream, chilled overnight

2 tsp (10 ml) maple syrup

1 tsp cinnamon

Now, we'll make our whipped topping. I recommend chilling your mixing bowl and whisk attachment beater in the freezer for at least 10 minutes before beginning the whipped topping steps. This will help the whipped topping form quicker.

Add the chilled coconut cream, maple syrup, and cinnamon to the bowl of a stand mixer and beat it with the whisk attachment for 4 to 5 minutes, until it's nice and fluffy. Spread the whipped topping on your pie just before serving.

Store the pie covered in the refrigerator (without the whipped topping) for up to 1 week. Store the whipped topping in a separate container for up to 5 days.

TIPS: This is not an overly sweet pie. The layers combine together perfectly for a subtly sweet pie with a hint of saltiness from the crust. But, if you would like a more intense sweet flavor, add a couple tablespoons (30 ml) more of maple syrup to the filling—just remember you'll need to adjust the nutrition information provided accordingly.

For an extra special touch, top it off with some toasted coconut flakes too!

Nutrition Info (Serving size: $1/16$ of pie): Calories: 255, Total Fat: 17 g, Saturated Fat: 9 g, Total Carbohydrates: 21 g, Sugar: 14 g, Fiber: 3 g, Sodium: 68 mg, Protein: 7 g

funfetti® birthday cake

Yes, you can manage your blood sugars and enjoy your cake too! The fun pop of sprinkles in this birthday cake pairs perfectly with my go-to blood sugar–friendly combo of oats and almond flour. And a lower-sugar glaze gives you that perfect cake flavor without packing on the excess sugar that comes with traditional frosting.

high protein | yield: 16 pieces

⅓ cup (80 ml) unsweetened applesauce

⅓ cup (76 ml) unsalted butter, melted

2 large eggs, beaten

⅓ cup (80 ml) agave syrup

¼ cup (60 ml) avocado oil

3 tsp (15 ml) vanilla extract, divided

2 cups (190 g) almond flour

1¼ cups (113 g) rolled oats, ground

1 tsp baking soda

½ tsp baking powder

2 tbsp (24 g) rainbow sprinkles

1 tbsp (14 g) softened butter

2 tbsp (30 ml) whole milk

1 cup (120 g) powdered sugar, sifted

Preheat your oven to 350°F (177°C). Grease two 8-inch (20-cm) cake pans and set them aside.

In a medium-sized mixing bowl, combine the applesauce, butter, eggs, agave, avocado oil, and 2 teaspoons (10 ml) of vanilla extract. Whisk them together until well combined. Set that bowl aside.

Now, in another medium-sized mixing bowl, mix together the almond flour, ground oats, baking soda, and baking powder until just combined. Add these dry ingredients to the bowl with your wet ingredients and mix until everything is combined and you don't see any dry ingredients remaining. Gently stir in the sprinkles.

Divide the batter evenly between the two greased cake pans. Place the cakes in the oven and bake for 15 to 20 minutes, or until a toothpick inserted in the center of the cake comes out clean. Let the cakes cool completely before removing them from the cake pans.

To make the glaze, in a bowl, combine the remaining 1 teaspoon of vanilla extract, 1 tablespoon (14 g) of softened butter, and whole milk and whisk to fully combine. Slowly add the powdered sugar to the bowl and whisk as you go until a nice, slightly runny glaze has formed.

Stack your two round cakes on top of each other and pour the glaze on the top of the cake. Slice and enjoy!

You can store your cakes (without the glaze) in the freezer for up to 6 months. Just make sure they're wrapped well in plastic wrap or foil to prevent freezer burn. Once you add the glaze to the cake, you can store any leftovers in the refrigerator for up to 7 days in a sealed container.

Nutrition Info (Serving size: 1 slice): Calories: 228, Total Fat: 15 g, Saturated Fat: 4.5 g, Total Carbohydrates: 19 g, Sugar: 12 g, Fiber: 2 g, Sodium: 105 mg, Protein: 5 g

TIP: If you want to really wow with your presentation, double the recipe and build a four-layer cake!

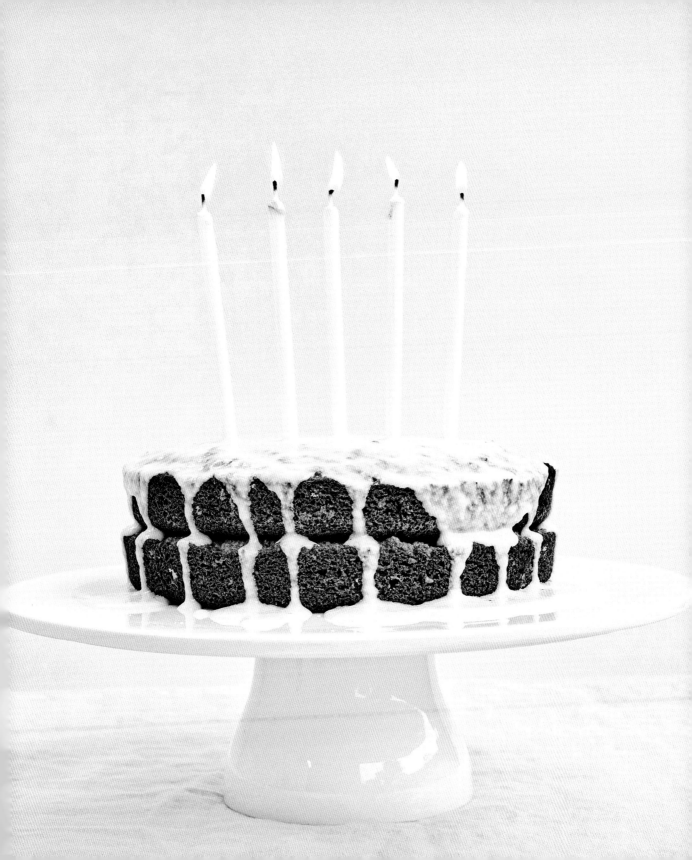

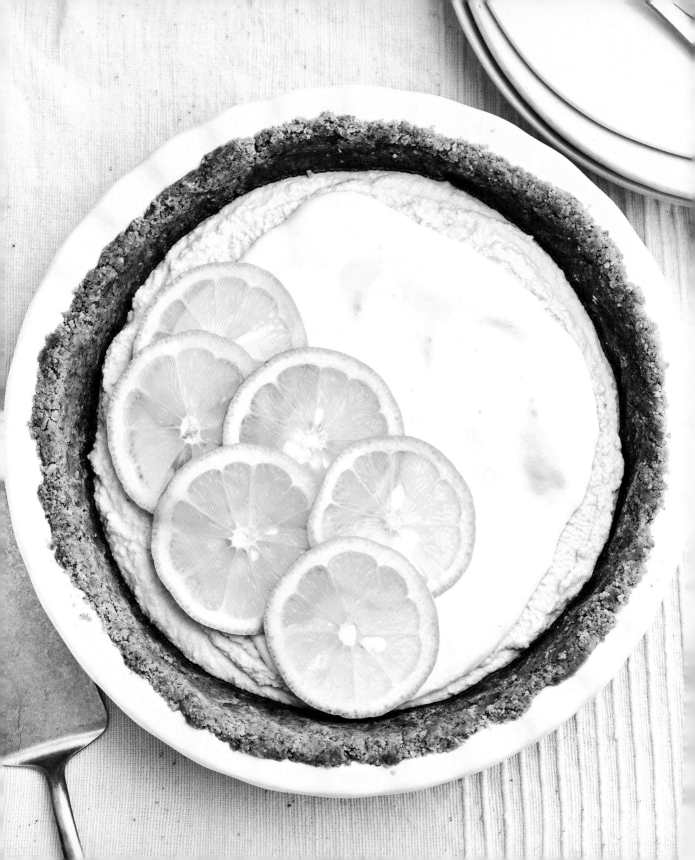

simple lemon icebox pie

Nothing is more refreshing on a hot day than a slice of classic lemon icebox pie! So, to make this version a bit more blood sugar friendly, we've swapped the sweetened condensed milk for evaporated milk and are adding the sweetener ourselves. This way, we can control how much sugar we're adding in and prevent any blood sugar spikes later on.

high fiber | high protein | yield: 12 slices

CRUST

1 cup (95 g) almond flour

1 cup (90 g) rolled oats

¼ cup (50 g) coconut sugar

4 tbsp (57 g) unsalted butter, melted

FILLING

8 oz (224 g) low-fat cream cheese, softened

12 oz (336 ml) low-fat evaporated milk

¼ cup (60 ml) lemon juice

Zest from ½ of a lemon (6 g)

¼ cup (60 ml) agave nectar, or other preferred liquid sweetener

1 cup (120 g) coconut flour

TOPPING

1 cup (40 g) whipped cream

6 round lemon slices

To the bowl of a food processor or blender, add the almond flour, oats, coconut sugar, and melted butter. Process them all together until the mixture resembles wet sand, 15 to 20 seconds. Then, carefully transfer the mixture to an 8- or 9-inch (20- or 23-cm) pie plate and press it down and up the sides.

Now for the filling! We're going to use the food processor or blender again, so give it a quick rinse and dry. Then add your cream cheese, evaporated milk, lemon juice, lemon zest, agave nectar, and coconut flour to the food processor and process for 15 to 20 seconds, until a smooth mixture forms. Pour the filling into the pie crust and refrigerate for at least 4 hours to allow it to set and firm up.

Before serving, top it off with the whipped cream and garnish with the lemon slices.

Store the pie covered in your refrigerator for up to 1 week, or freeze for up to 6 months.

> TIP: There are so many different ways you can adapt this recipe depending on your preferences or what ingredients you have on hand! Make sure to check out the substitution chart on page 16 if you're missing an ingredient!

Nutrition Info (Serving size: 1 slice): Calories: 255, Total Fat: 15 g, Saturated Fat: 7 g, Total Carbohydrates: 29 g, Sugar: 17 g, Fiber: 7 g, Sodium: 127 mg, Protein: 7 g

classic pumpkin pie

Classic pumpkin pie gets a blood sugar–friendly makeover in this traditionally delicious pumpkin pie recipe! The crust is balanced out with almond flour and oats, and we've cut back on the sugar content by using evaporated milk instead of the traditional sweetened condensed milk. You'll never make any other pumpkin pie recipe again!

high protein | yield: 16 slices

CRUST

1½ cups (146 g) almond flour

3 tbsp (18 g) rolled oats

3 tbsp (45 g) granulated sugar

3 tbsp (42 g) butter, softened

1 large egg

½ tsp ground cinnamon

FILLING

1 (15-oz [425-g]) can pumpkin puree

3 large eggs

¼ cup (60 ml) pure maple syrup

¼ cup (50 g) granulated sugar

⅓ cup (80 ml) evaporated milk

½ tsp vanilla extract

½ tsp almond extract

1 tsp cinnamon

½ tsp nutmeg

1 tsp ground ginger

½ tsp salt

Preheat your oven to 350°F (177°C) and grease a 9-inch (23-cm) pie plate (or a deep dish 8-inch [20-cm] pie plate) well with butter or cooking spray. Set the pie plate aside.

First, we're going to prepare our crust. To the bowl of a large food processor, add the almond flour, oats, sugar, butter, egg, and cinnamon. Process the ingredients until a dough ball has formed, about 10 seconds. Then, carefully transfer the mixture to your greased pie plate. Press the mixture down into the bottom of the pan and all the way up the sides of your pie plate. Bake the pie crust for 13 to 14 minutes, just until it starts to turn golden brown.

While the crust is baking, in a bowl, combine the pumpkin puree, eggs, maple syrup, sugar, evaporated milk, vanilla extract, almond extract, cinnamon, nutmeg, ginger, and salt. Whisk them together until smooth. Pour the filling into the baked pie crust. Return the pie to the oven and bake for 60 to 75 minutes, or until the center of the pie is set and only slightly jiggly.

Store your pie covered in the refrigerator for up to 1 week.

> TIP: If the edges of your pie crust start to get too dark while baking, remove the pie from the oven and cover the edges with foil. Return the pie to the oven to finish baking.

Nutrition Info (Serving size: 1 slice): Calories: 166, Total Fat: 8 g, Saturated Fat: 2 g, Total Carbohydrates: 19 g, Sugar: 9 g, Fiber: 4 g, Sodium: 151 mg, Protein: 5 g

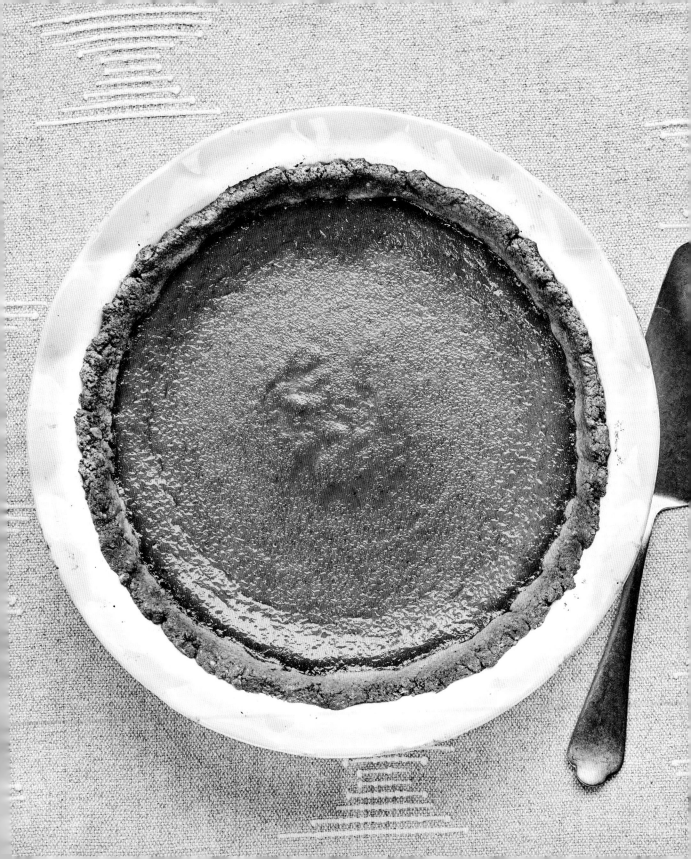

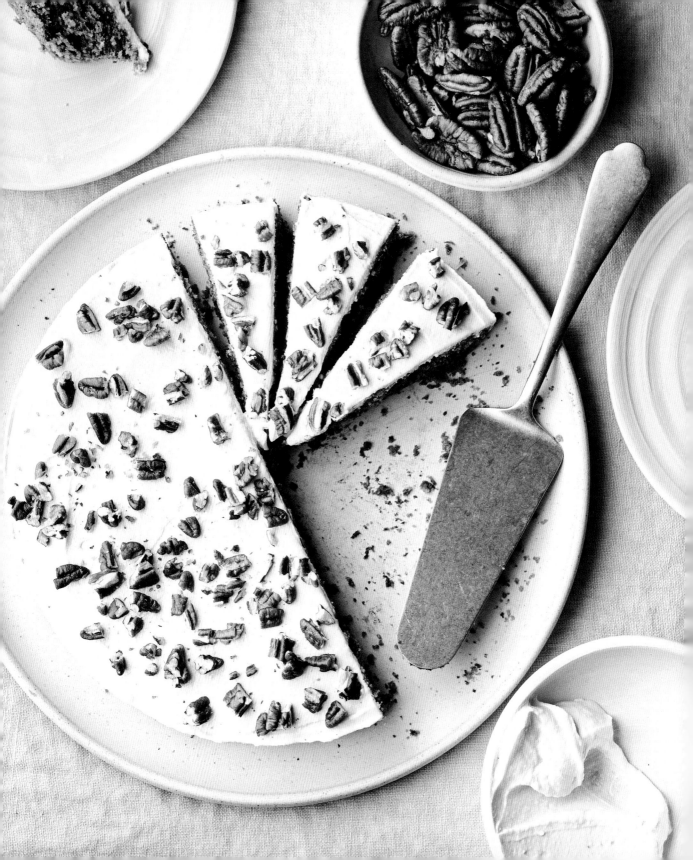

carrot spice cake with greek yogurt icing

Classic carrot cake gets a blood sugar makeover in this recipe! My go-to combo of oats and almond flour makes a fluffy cake. We add in hints of spice and raisins for a classic carrot cake flavor but with less sugar. And of course, we can't go without some lower-sugar cream cheese frosting!

high protein | yield: 16 slices

CAKE

⅓ cup (80 ml) unsweetened applesauce

⅓ cup (76 ml) unsalted butter, melted

2 large eggs, beaten

⅓ cup (80 ml) maple syrup

¼ cup (60 ml) avocado oil

2 tsp (10 ml) vanilla extract

2 cups (190 g) almond flour

1¼ cups (113 g) rolled oats, ground

1 tsp baking soda

½ tsp baking powder

2 tsp (5 g) cinnamon

1 tsp ginger

1 tsp nutmeg

½ tsp cloves

½ cup (55 g) shredded carrots

½ cup (54 g) pecan pieces, divided

Preheat your oven to 350°F (177°C). Grease an 8- or 9-inch (20- or 23-cm) cake pan and set it aside.

In a medium-sized mixing bowl, combine the applesauce, butter, eggs, maple syrup, avocado oil, and vanilla extract. Whisk them together until well combined. Set that bowl aside.

Now, in another medium-sized mixing bowl, mix together the almond flour, ground oats, baking soda, baking powder, cinnamon, ginger, nutmeg, and cloves until just combined. Add these dry ingredients to the bowl with your wet ingredients and mix until everything is combined and you don't see any dry ingredients remaining. Gently stir in the shredded carrots, and ¼ cup (27 g) of the pecan pieces.

Add the batter to your greased pan. Place the cake in the oven and bake for 20 to 25 minutes, or until a toothpick inserted in the center of the cake comes out clean.

Let the cake cool completely before removing it from the cake pan.

(continued)

carrot spice cake with greek yogurt icing (cont.)

ICING

4 oz (112 g) low-fat cream cheese, softened

½ cup (120 ml) plain whole milk Greek yogurt

2 tbsp (15 g) coconut flour

2 tbsp (30 ml) maple syrup

½ tsp vanilla extract

To make the icing, combine the cream cheese, Greek yogurt, coconut flour, maple syrup, and vanilla extract. Mix it together fully until smooth.

Spread a thin layer of icing on the top and sides of the cake. Sprinkle with the remaining ¼ cup (27 g) of pecan pieces. Slice and enjoy!

You can store your cake (without the icing) in the freezer for up to 6 months. Just make sure it's wrapped well in plastic wrap or foil to prevent freezer burn. Once you add the icing to the cake, you can store any leftovers in the refrigerator for up to 7 days in a sealed container.

TIP: If you want to really wow with your presentation, double the recipe and build a layer cake!

Nutrition Info (Serving size: 1 slice): Calories: 250, Total Fat: 18 g, Saturated Fat: 5 g, Total Carbohydrates: 16 g, Sugar: 8 g, Fiber: 3 g, Sodium: 143 mg, Protein: 7 g

key lime cupcakes with yogurt icing

Whether it's a birthday party, a summer barbecue, or any special occasion, who doesn't love a good cupcake? These are packed with huge flavor thanks to almond extract and key lime zest. These cupcakes are a deliciously blood sugar–friendly way to satisfy your sweet tooth!

high protein | quick & simple | yield: 18 cupcakes

CUPCAKES

⅓ cup (80 ml) unsweetened applesauce

⅓ cup (76 g) unsalted butter, melted

2 large eggs, beaten

⅓ cup (80 ml) agave syrup

¼ cup (60 ml) avocado oil

1 tsp vanilla extract

¼ cup (60 ml) key lime juice

½ tbsp (3 g) key lime zest

2 cups (190 g) almond flour

1½ cups (135 g) rolled oats, ground

1 tsp baking soda

½ tsp baking powder

Preheat your oven to 350°F (177°C). Grease 18 muffin/cupcake wells, or use liners. Set the pan aside.

In a medium-sized mixing bowl, combine the applesauce, butter, eggs, agave, avocado oil, vanilla extract, key lime juice, and key lime zest. Whisk them together until well combined. Set that bowl aside.

Now, in another medium-sized mixing bowl, mix together the almond flour, oats, baking soda, and baking powder until just combined. Add these dry ingredients to the bowl with your wet ingredients and mix until everything is combined and you don't see any dry ingredients remaining.

Pour your batter evenly into the 18 muffin/cupcake wells. Place the pans in the oven and bake for 15 to 20 minutes, or until a toothpick inserted in the center comes out clean.

Let the cupcakes cool completely before removing them from the pans.

(continued)

key lime cupcakes with yogurt icing (cont.)

ICING

1 cup (240 ml) plain whole milk Greek yogurt

¼ cup (30 g) coconut flour

2 tbsp (30 ml) agave syrup

½ tsp vanilla extract

1 tbsp (15 ml) key lime juice

½ tbsp (3 g) key lime zest

While they cool, we can mix up our icing. In a bowl, add the Greek yogurt, coconut flour, agave syrup, vanilla extract, key lime juice, and key lime zest to a bowl. Whisk them together until well combined.

Once the cupcakes have cooled completely, you can spread or pipe the icing on top. Sprinkle with some additional key lime zest or garnish with key lime wheels and enjoy!

Store your cupcakes (without icing) in the freezer in a sealed container for up to 6 months. Once iced, cupcakes will keep for 3 days in the refrigerator in a sealed container.

TIP: The icing in this recipe also makes a great fruit dip! Try dipping your favorites in it for a refreshing snack!

Nutrition Info (Serving size: 1 cupcake with icing): Calories: 200, Total Fat: 13 g, Saturated Fat: 4 g, Total Carbohydrates: 15 g, Sugar: 7 g, Fiber: 3 g, Sodium: 99 mg, Protein: 6 g

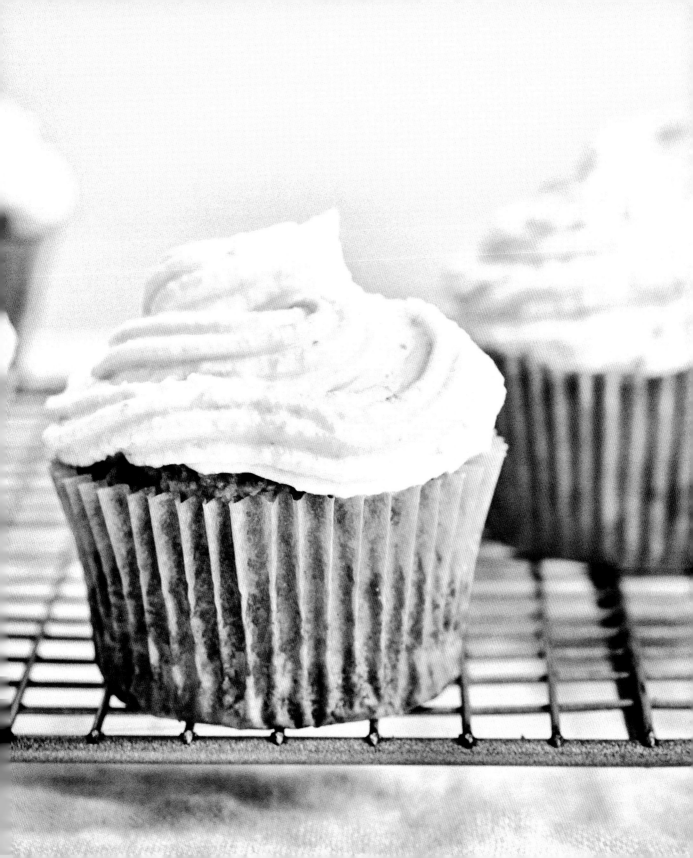

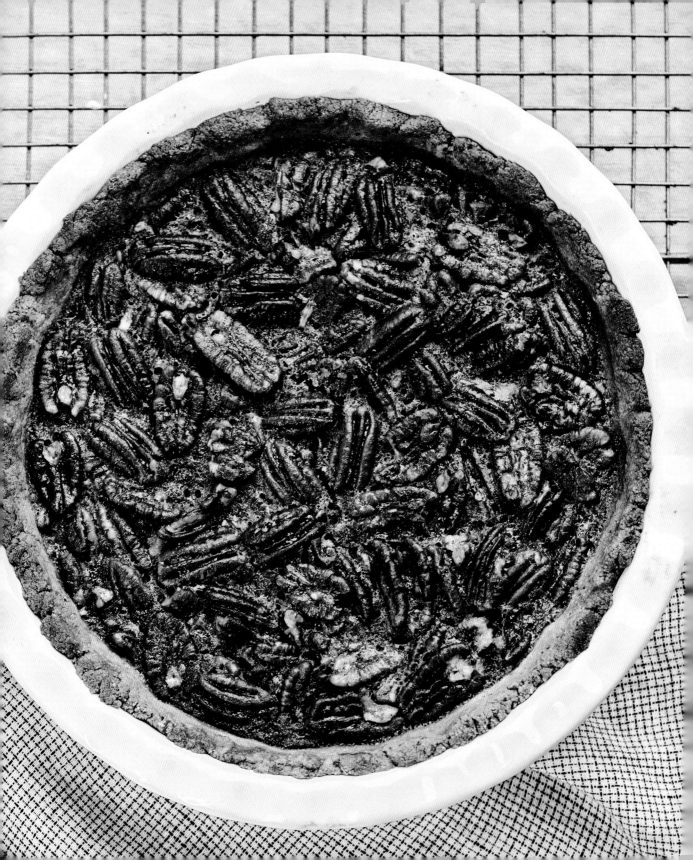

maple pecan pie with almond flour crust

If you've ever turned down a slice of pecan pie during the holiday season because you were afraid it had too much sugar, you must try this recipe! The blood sugar–friendly crust and a reduced-sugar filling combined with better-for-you plant-based fats and protein from the pecans make this one dessert you can always say yes to!

gluten-free | high protein | yield: 16 slices

CRUST

1¾ cups (166 g) + 2 tbsp (12 g) almond flour

3 tbsp (39 g) coconut sugar

3 tbsp (42 g) unsalted butter, softened

1 large egg

FILLING

½ cup (120 ml) maple syrup

4 oz (120 ml) evaporated milk

3 large eggs, beaten

¼ cup (50 g) coconut sugar

1½ tsp (8 ml) vanilla extract

2 tbsp (28 g) unsalted butter, melted

2 cups (218 g) pecan halves

Preheat your oven to 350°F (177°C). Grease a 9-inch (23-cm) pie plate (or a deep dish 8-inch [20-cm] pie plate) well with butter or cooking spray. Set the pie plate aside.

To the bowl of a large food processor, add the almond flour, coconut sugar, softened butter, and egg. Process the ingredients until a dough ball has formed, about 10 seconds. Then, carefully transfer the mixture to your greased pie plate. Press the mixture down into the bottom of the pan and all the way up the sides of your pie plate. Bake the pie crust for 13 to 14 minutes, until it starts to turn golden brown.

While the pie crust is baking, in a bowl, mix together the maple syrup, evaporated milk, eggs, coconut sugar, vanilla extract, melted butter, and pecans. Once the pie crust has finished baking, pour the pecan mixture into the pie crust.

Place the pie back in the oven and bake your pecan pie for 50 to 60 minutes, or until the center has started to set and the crust is golden brown.

Let the pie cool for at least 2 hours before cutting into it.

Store your pie in the refrigerator, covered, for up to 7 days. You can also store your pie tightly covered in the freezer for up to 3 months.

TIP: If the edges of your pie crust start to get too dark while baking, remove the pie from the oven and cover the edges with foil. Return the pie to the oven to finish baking.

Nutrition Info (Serving size: 1 slice): Calories: 262, Total Fat: 19 g, Saturated Fat: 4 g, Total Carbohydrates: 17 g, Sugar: 13 g, Fiber: 3 g, Sodium: 27 mg, Protein: 7 g

blueberry basil greek yogurt pie with cashew crust

This no-bake pie is the perfect make-ahead dessert with a unique flavor profile! And it's pretty easy on the eyes too! With 6 grams of fiber and 9 grams of protein per slice, you'll be satisfied and your blood sugars will be happy!

high fiber | high protein | yield: 12 slices

CRUST

¾ cup (71 g) almond flour

¾ cup (68 g) rolled oats

¼ cup (50 g) coconut sugar

⅓ cup (86 g) unsweetened cashew butter

FILLING

8 oz (224 g) low-fat cream cheese, softened

1 cup (240 ml) plain Greek yogurt

2 tbsp (30 ml) lemon juice

¼ cup (60 ml) agave nectar

¾ cup (90 g) coconut flour

2 tbsp (4 g) roughly chopped basil leaves

1 cup (148 g) frozen blueberries, thawed

To the bowl of a food processor, add the almond flour, oats, coconut sugar, and cashew butter. Process them all together until the mixture resembles wet sand, 15 to 20 seconds. Then, carefully transfer the mixture to an 8- or 9-inch (20- or 23-cm) pie plate and press it down and up the sides.

For the filling, we're going to use the food processor again, so give it a quick rinse and dry. Then, add your cream cheese, Greek yogurt, lemon juice, agave nectar, coconut flour, and basil leaves to the clean bowl of the food processor and process for 15 to 20 seconds, until a smooth mixture forms. Remove the blade from the food processor and carefully stir in your thawed blueberries. I love the pretty purple/blue streaks they make! Pour the filling into the pie crust and refrigerate for at least 4 hours to allow it to set and firm up.

Store your pie in the refrigerator covered for up to 1 week.

TIPS: I know it may seem odd to use thawed frozen blueberries here. Why can't we just use fresh blueberries? The reason why is that the juice that is produced when you thaw blueberries that were previously frozen adds to the texture of the pie and gives those pretty blue/purple streaks!

If you like this pie, make sure to try the Simple Lemon Icebox Pie (page 69). It's equally as simple to make and equally delicious!

Nutrition Info (Serving size: 1 slice): Calories: 218, Total Fat: 12 g, Saturated Fat: 4 g, Total Carbohydrates: 25 g, Sugar: 14 g, Fiber: 6 g, Sodium: 102 mg, Protein: 9 g

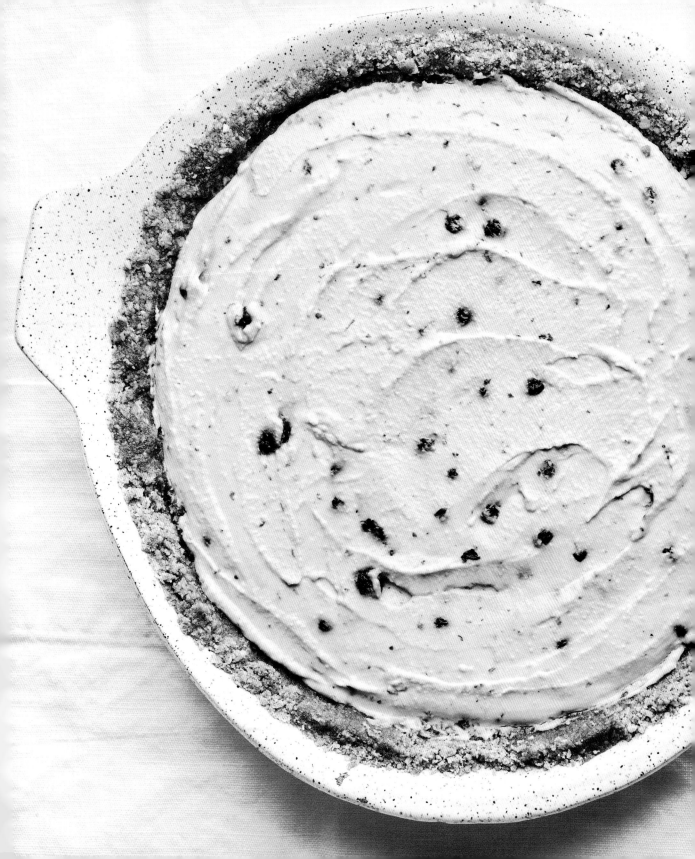

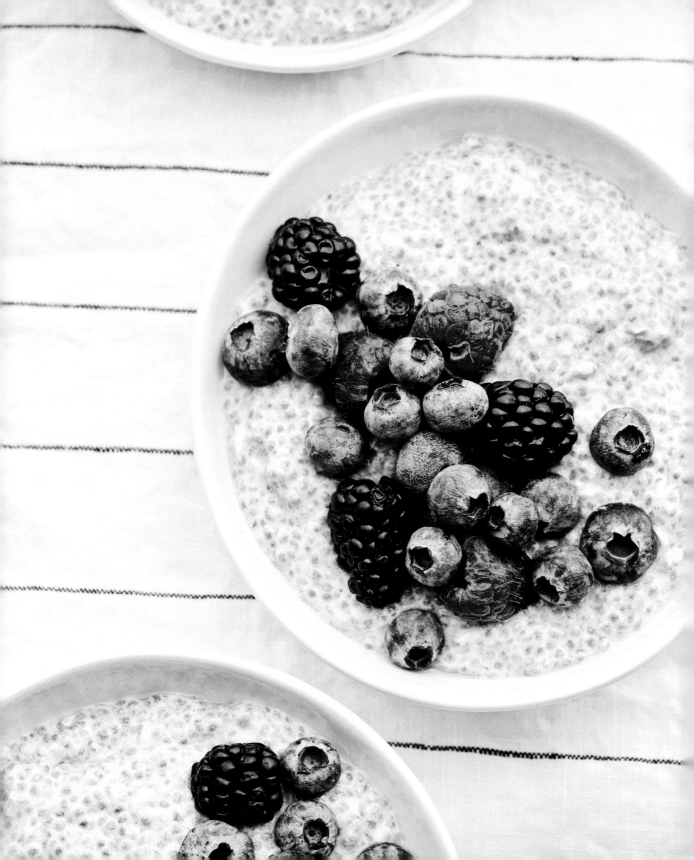

dessert for breakfast

I'm fairly certain every kid at some point in their life has dreamed of getting to eat dessert for breakfast every day . . . but then at some point we grow up and realize that that's maybe not the best way to start the day.

A blood sugar–balancing breakfast should have three things:

- A decent amount of fiber
- A quality source of protein
- Minimal added sugar

A quick look at the breakfast aisle in your local grocery store will show you that most of the packaged breakfast options available today don't have these. But, the beauty of making blood sugar–balancing desserts is that they meet all three of those criteria and can also be a great start to your day! So, we can have dessert for breakfast after all!

So, while my Classic Blueberry Banana Bread (page 87) could totally satisfy a sweet tooth after dinner, it can also get you going in the morning and keep blood sugars stable thanks to the fiber and protein content. And you have to try The Easiest Healthy Cinnamon Rolls (page 84). Like most of the recipes in this book, we cut back on the sugar slightly and use more nutrient-dense flours for a perfectly blood sugar–friendly option . . . and yes, they even still have a delicious icing on top!

the easiest healthy cinnamon rolls

These cinnamon rolls utilize a high-fiber, high-protein flour mix to create an easy batter for delicious cinnamon rolls without the crash. Lightly sweetened Greek yogurt serves in place of frosting for a creamy protein boost. The recipe comes together in less than 20 minutes, which makes baking cinnamon rolls much less intimidating!

gluten-free | high fiber | high protein | quick & simple | yield: 6 cinnamon rolls

1 large egg

¼ cup (60 ml) unsweetened almond milk

¾ cup (71 g) almond flour (plus some extra for flouring the rolling surface)

½ cup (60 g) tapioca flour

¼ cup (30 g) coconut flour

1 tbsp (8 g) cinnamon

1 tbsp (14 g) coconut oil, melted

2 tbsp (30 ml) maple syrup, divided

¼ cup (60 ml) plain nonfat Greek yogurt

½ tsp vanilla extract

Preheat your oven to 350°F (177°C). Grease a round baking dish and set it aside.

In a large mixing bowl, whisk together the egg and almond milk. Next, add the almond flour, tapioca flour, and coconut flour to the bowl and stir it together until a thick dough forms.

Now, dust some extra flour on a piece of parchment paper on your counter and roll out your dough approximately ½ inch (1.3 cm) thick.

In a separate small bowl, mix together the cinnamon, melted coconut oil, and 1 tablespoon (15 ml) of the maple syrup. Brush the mixture on the rolled out dough.

Then, dust your hands with flour and roll the dough into a long log. Using a sharp knife, make five slices to create six evenly sized cinnamon rolls and arrange them in a flat layer in the prepared baking dish.

Bake the cinnamon rolls for 8 to 10 minutes, or until the tops are slightly browned.

While they are baking, it's time to make the frosting. Whisk together the remaining 1 tablespoon (15 ml) of maple syrup, Greek yogurt, and vanilla extract. Once the rolls have been removed from the oven, drizzle the frosting across the tops and enjoy!

Store your cinnamon rolls covered in the fridge for up to 3 days.

TIP: A grain-free or Paleo pancake mix can be used in place of the almond flour, tapioca flour, and coconut flour.

Nutrition Info (Serving size: 1 cinnamon roll): Calories: 180, Total Fat: 9 g, Saturated Fat: 3 g, Total Carbohydrates: 21 g, Sugar: 6 g, Fiber: 5 g, Sodium: 30 mg, Protein: 7 g

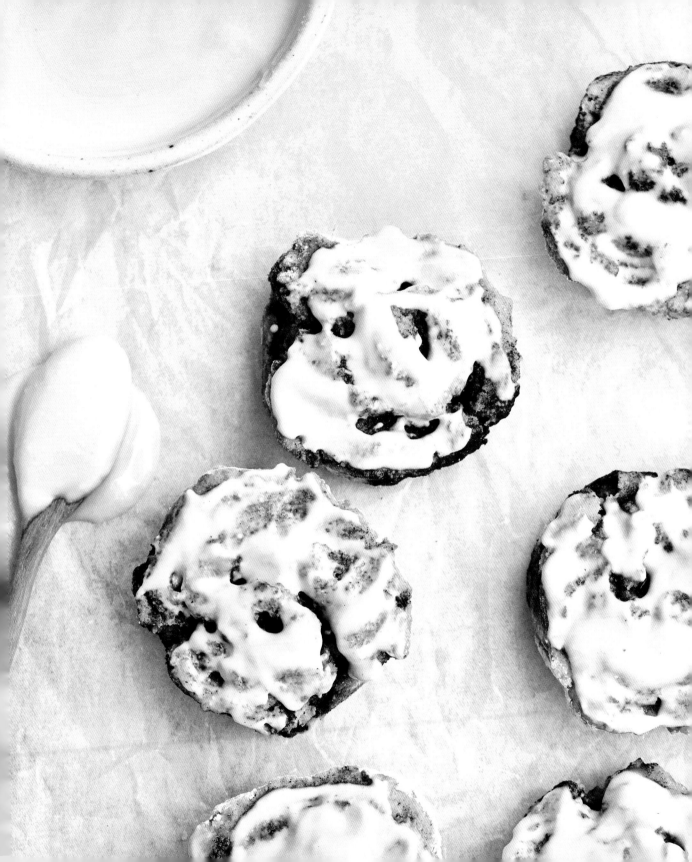

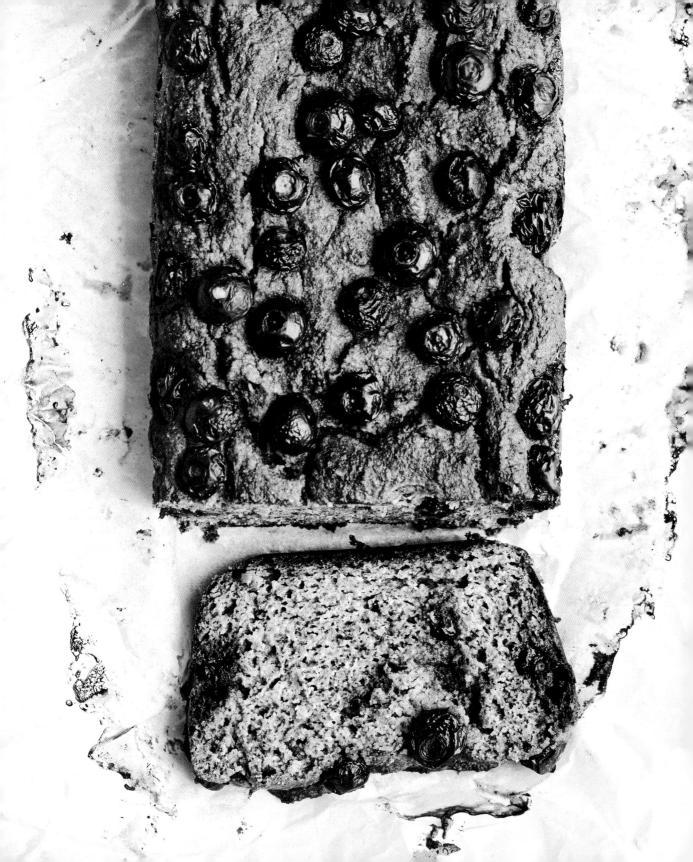

classic blueberry banana bread

Bananas get a bad rap for people with diabetes, but fear not! These delicious fruits have 3 grams of fiber each, plus important nutrients like potassium, vitamin B6, vitamin C, and magnesium. In this recipe, we pair bananas with healthy fats and protein from almond flour, flax seeds, almond butter, and Greek yogurt to create a delicious, blood sugar–friendly breakfast treat.

gluten-free | high protein | yield: 12 servings

1 cup (95 g) almond flour

¼ cup (30 g) coconut flour

¼ cup (28 g) ground flax seeds

1 tsp cinnamon

1 tsp baking powder

½ tsp baking soda

Pinch of salt

3 large eggs

3 mashed bananas, about 1 cup (225 g)

2 tbsp (32 g) almond butter

¼ cup (60 ml) maple syrup

½ cup (120 ml) plain Greek yogurt

1 tsp vanilla extract

1 cup (148 g) blueberries, divided

First, preheat the oven to 350°F (177°C). Line a loaf pan with parchment paper. Be sure to leave some overhang so you can easily pull the baked loaf out of the pan when it's done baking. Set the loaf pan aside.

Now, in a large mixing bowl, combine the almond flour, coconut flour, ground flax seeds, cinnamon, baking powder, baking soda, and salt. In a second mixing bowl, whisk the eggs and then add the mashed bananas, almond butter, maple syrup, Greek yogurt, and vanilla extract. Combine the dry and wet ingredients and mix them together. There will be some lumps and that's okay.

Pour half the batter into the lined loaf pan, add in ½ cup (74 g) of the blueberries, then add the remaining batter and top with the remaining blueberries. Bake the bread for 55 to 60 minutes, or until a toothpick inserted into the center comes out clean.

Allow the bread to cool for 20 to 30 minutes before slicing it.

Store in an airtight container on the counter for 1 to 2 days, in the fridge for up to 7 days, or in the freezer for 6 months.

TIP: Freeze leftover banana bread after slicing for an easy breakfast you can reheat in no time!

Nutrition Info (Serving size: 1 slice): Calories: 169, Total Fat: 9 g, Saturated Fat: 1 g, Total Carbohydrates: 18 g, Sugar: 10 g, Fiber: 4 g, Sodium: 233 mg, Protein: 6 g

3-in-1 breakfast cookies

Craving a portable and sweet breakfast without the sugar crash? With 1 simple base recipe and 3 flavor variations, these high-protein breakfast cookies are sure to please the whole family and keep energy levels and blood sugars nice and stable.

dairy-free | high protein | quick & simple | yield: 8 cookies

BASE RECIPE

2 tbsp (27 ml) coconut oil, melted

2 large eggs

2 tbsp (32 g) almond butter

1½ tbsp (23 ml) maple syrup

½ tsp vanilla extract

½ cup (48 g) almond flour

1 cup (90 g) rolled oats

¼ cup (28 g) ground flax seeds

FLAVOR OPTION #1: GRANOLA

½ cup (45 g) granola

FLAVOR OPTION #2: WHITE CHOCOLATE RASPBERRY

¼ cup (42 g) white chocolate chips

¼ cup (5 g) freeze-dried raspberries

FLAVOR OPTION #3: CARROT CAKE

1 carrot, grated (about ⅓ cup [15 g])

2 Medjool dates, pitted and chopped

¼ cup (29 g) walnuts, crushed

½ tsp cinnamon

Preheat your oven to 350°F (177°C). Line a baking sheet with parchment paper and set it aside.

In a large mixing bowl, whisk together the melted coconut oil, eggs, almond butter, maple syrup, and vanilla extract.

In a separate mixing bowl, add the almond flour, oats, and flax seeds. Then, combine these two mixtures and mix until smooth.

Now, add in the mix-ins for the flavor variation you want to make.

Next, use a cookie scoop to drop the batter onto the prepared baking sheet. Bake for 10 to 12 minutes, or until the edges are lightly browned. Let the cookies cool completely on a wire rack before storing.

Store in an airtight container for up to a week in the refrigerator or freeze for up to 3 months.

TIP: Freeze-dried fruit is a great add-in for baking because it won't add unnecessary moisture to the batter. (Extra moisture can lead to cookies that just won't bake.) Be sure to look for unsweetened varieties.

Nutrition Info

Granola (Serving size: 1 cookie): Calories: 211, Total Fat: 14 g, Saturated Fat: 4 g, Total Carbohydrates: 17 g, Sugar: 4 g, Fiber: 3 g, Sodium: 104 mg, Protein: 7 g

White Chocolate Raspberry (Serving size: 1 cookie): Calories: 211, Total Fat: 13 g, Saturated Fat: 6 g, Total Carbohydrates: 19 g, Sugar: 7 g, Fiber: 3 g, Sodium: 71 mg, Protein: 5 g

Carrot Cake (Serving size: 1 cookie): Calories: 220, Total Fat: 14 g, Saturated Fat: 4 g, Total Carbohydrates: 18 g, Sugar: 6 g, Fiber: 4 g, Sodium: 85 mg, Protein: 7 g

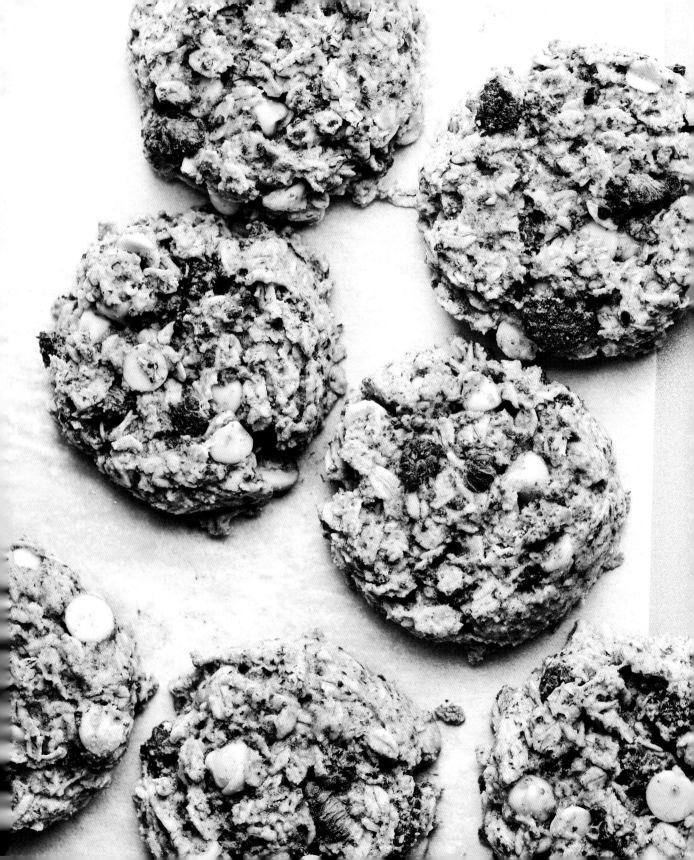

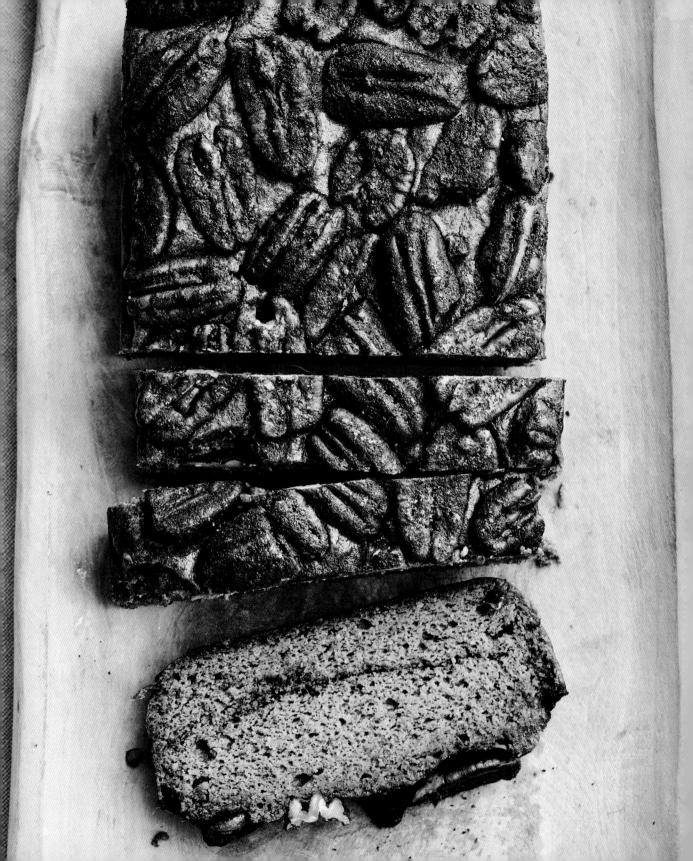

low-carb pumpkin bread

Classic pumpkin bread gets a makeover with high-fiber coconut flour as the base. The batter is generously spiced with warming fall flavors, almond and vanilla extracts, and toasted spiced pecans. The fragrant flavor profile helps keep the sugar content low without sacrificing taste.

dairy-free | gluten-free | yield: 10 slices

3 large eggs

¼ cup (65 g) almond butter

6 tbsp (90 ml) maple syrup, divided

1 cup (244 g) canned pumpkin puree

¼ cup (60 ml) avocado oil

2 tsp (10 ml) vanilla extract

2 tsp (10 ml) almond extract

¼ cup (30 g) coconut flour

1 tbsp (8 g) + 2 tsp (5 g) cinnamon, divided

1 tbsp (8 g) pumpkin pie spice

1 tsp baking powder

Pinch of sea salt

1 tbsp (14 g) coconut oil, melted

½ cup (55 g) pecan halves

Start by preheating your oven to 350°F (177°C). Line a loaf pan with parchment paper and set it aside.

In a food processor or blender, mix the eggs, almond butter, 5 tablespoons (75 ml) of the maple syrup, pumpkin puree, avocado oil, vanilla extract, and almond extract until smooth.

In a separate bowl, whisk the coconut flour, 2 teaspoons (5 g) of cinnamon, pumpkin pie spice, baking powder, and salt. Pour the wet ingredient mixture into the bowl of dry ingredients. Mix them together until combined. Set this batter aside.

Now, in a small dish, add the melted coconut oil, the remaining 1 tablespoon (15 ml) of maple syrup, and remaining 1 tablespoon (8 g) of cinnamon. Whisk these together until combined and set it aside.

In a parchment-lined loaf pan, add your ingredients in the following order:

* Half of the batter
* Half of the coconut oil, cinnamon, and maple syrup mixture
* Remaining half of the batter

Then, stir the pecan halves into the remaining coconut oil mixture and mix until the pecans are coated. Top the loaf with the coated pecan halves.

Bake the bread for 55 minutes, or until an inserted toothpick comes out clean.

Store your pumpkin bread in an airtight container on the counter for 1 to 2 days, in the fridge for up to 7 days, or in the freezer for 6 months.

Nutrition Info (Serving size: 1 slice): Calories: 213, Total Fat: 16 g, Saturated Fat: 3 g, Total Carbohydrates: 15 g, Sugar: 9 g, Fiber: 3 g, Sodium: 139 mg, Protein: 4 g

lean green zucchini bread

Mashed avocado replaces oil in this delicious zucchini bread! This not only adds to its distinct green hue, but also provides a hefty dose of fiber and healthy fats. Cinnamon, ginger, vanilla extract, and almond extract provide a natural sweetness, which help us keep the added sweetener to a minimum in this recipe.

dairy-free | gluten-free | high fiber | high protein | yield: 8 servings

1 cup (95 g) almond flour

¼ cup (30 g) coconut flour

½ tsp baking soda

1 tsp baking powder

1 tsp cinnamon

½ tsp ground ginger

Pinch of salt

1 cup (196 g) grated zucchini

3 large eggs

1 banana, mashed

2 tbsp (32 g) almond butter

1 medium avocado, peeled, pit removed, and mashed

⅓ cup (80 ml) maple syrup

1 tsp vanilla extract

½ tsp almond extract

Preheat your oven to 350°F (177°C). Line a loaf pan with parchment paper. Be sure to leave some overhang so you can easily pull the baked loaf out of the pan. Set the loaf pan aside.

In a large mixing bowl, combine the almond flour, coconut flour, baking soda, baking powder, cinnamon, ginger, and salt.

Next, we need to remove any excess water from our grated zucchini. Microwave it for 30 seconds and give it a good squeeze with a cheesecloth or dish towel.

Now, in a separate bowl, whisk the eggs and add the mashed banana, almond butter, mashed avocado, maple syrup, vanilla extract, almond extract, and grated zucchini. Then, slowly add the wet ingredients to the dry ingredients and mix together until well combined.

Finally, pour the batter into the loaf pan and bake the bread for 55 to 60 minutes, or until a toothpick inserted into the center comes out clean.

Let the bread cool for 20 to 30 minutes before slicing.

Store in an airtight container for up to 2 days, in the fridge for up to a week, or in the freezer for up to 3 months.

Nutrition info (Serving size: 1 slice): Calories: 214, Total Fat: 13 g, Saturated Fat: 2 g, Total Carbohydrates: 20 g, Sugar: 11 g, Fiber: 5 g, Sodium: 324 mg, Protein: 7 g

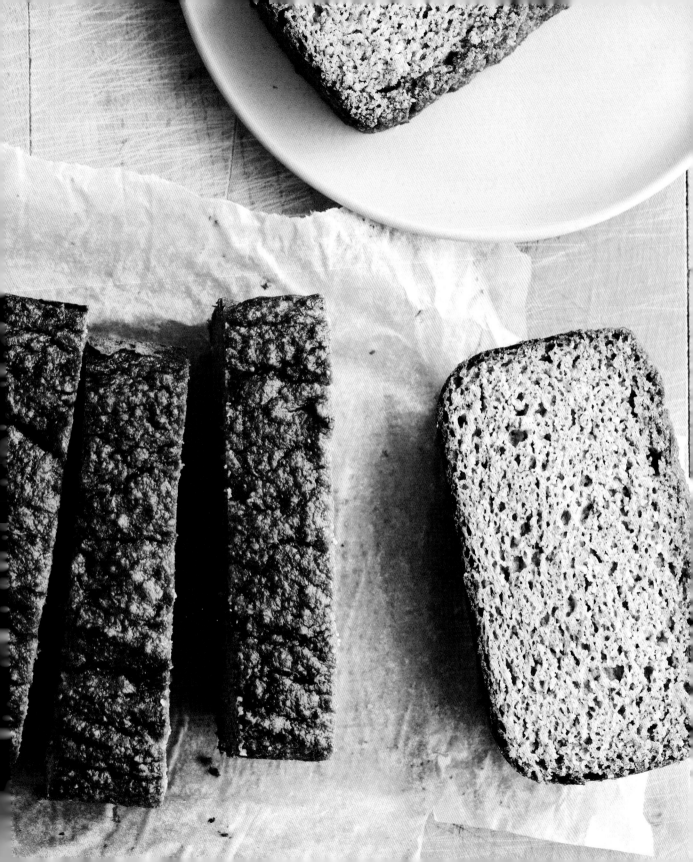

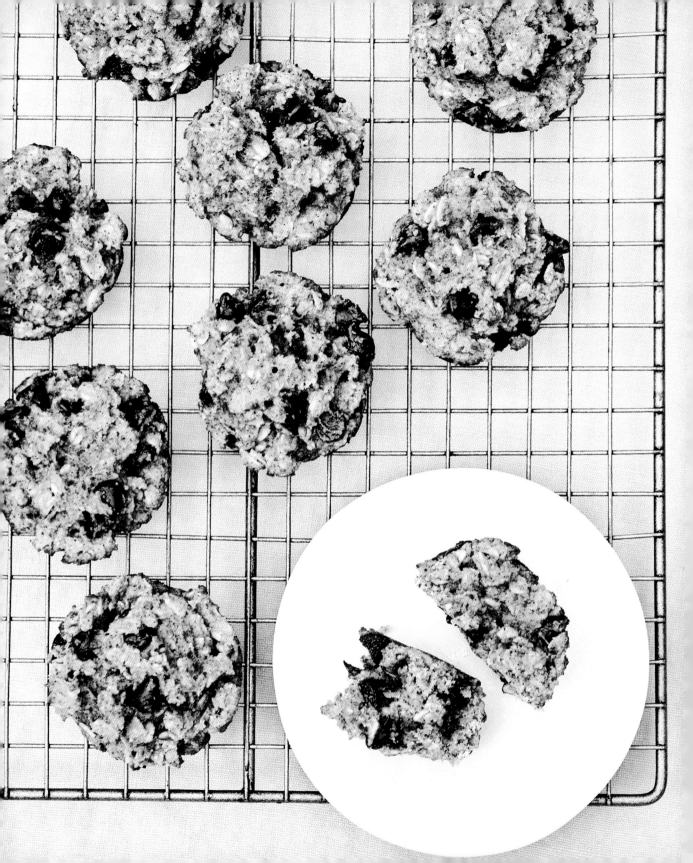

almond flour chocolate chip muffins

Almond flour and oats mimic the texture of classic bakery-style muffins, but with a protein and fiber upgrade! Almond butter and mashed banana keep these muffins moist and lightly sweet while adding an additional nutrient boost. These are the perfect grab-and-go breakfast to keep you satisfied and energized.

dairy-free | high protein | quick & simple | yield: 12 muffins

1 cup (95 g) almond flour

1 cup (90 g) rolled oats

1 tsp baking powder

1 tsp cinnamon

2 large eggs

¼ cup (65 g) almond butter

1 tsp vanilla extract

1½ bananas, mashed

½ cup (84 g) semi-sweet chocolate chips

Preheat your oven to 350°F (177°C). Grease a muffin tin and set it aside.

In a large mixing bowl, combine the almond flour, oats, baking powder, and cinnamon.

In a separate bowl, whisk the eggs, almond butter, vanilla extract, and mashed banana together well. Add these wet ingredients to the bowl with the dry ingredients and mix them all together. There will be some lumps, but that's okay!

Fold in the chocolate chips and pour the batter into the prepared muffin tin. Bake your muffins for 15 minutes, or until the tops are set and a toothpick comes out clean.

Store your muffins in an airtight container for up to 2 days, in the refrigerator for up to a week, or in the freezer for up to 3 months.

TIP: Feel free to substitute white chocolate chips or a dried fruit of choice for the semi-sweet chocolate chips. Just remember to update your nutritional information accordingly if needed.

Nutrition Info (Serving size: 1 muffin): Calories: 171, Total Fat: 11 g, Saturated Fat: 2 g, Total Carbohydrates: 16 g, Sugar: 6 g, Fiber: 3 g, Sodium: 54 mg, Protein: 5 g

creamy chia oatmeal pudding

Chia seeds are the star of this recipe. With 5 grams of fiber per tablespoon and heart-healthy omega-3 fats, chia is the perfect addition to your breakfast. They also expand up to ten times their size, creating a bouncy, pudding texture that's super blood sugar friendly!

high fiber | high protein | yield: 4 servings

1½ cups (360 ml) unsweetened almond milk

½ cup (120 ml) lemon juice

2 tsp (4 g) lemon zest

2 tsp (10 ml) vanilla extract

½ cup (120 ml) plain nonfat Greek yogurt

4 tsp (20 ml) maple syrup

½ cup (81 g) chia seeds

½ cup (45 g) rolled oats

In a large bowl, whisk together the almond milk, lemon juice, lemon zest, vanilla extract, yogurt, and maple syrup until smooth.

Next, stir in the chia seeds and oats until everything is well combined.

Cover and let it sit in the refrigerator for at least 4 hours or overnight before serving.

Keep your chia oatmeal pudding in an airtight jar in the fridge for 3 to 4 days.

TIP: If you prefer a creamier, more uniform texture, feel free to add the pudding to a blender and mix on high for 10 to 15 seconds before enjoying.

Nutrition Info (Serving size: ¼ of the recipe): Calories: 216, Total Fat: 10 g, Saturated Fat: 0 g, Total Carbohydrates: 27 g, Sugar: 8 g, Fiber: 8 g, Sodium: 68 mg, Protein: 7 g

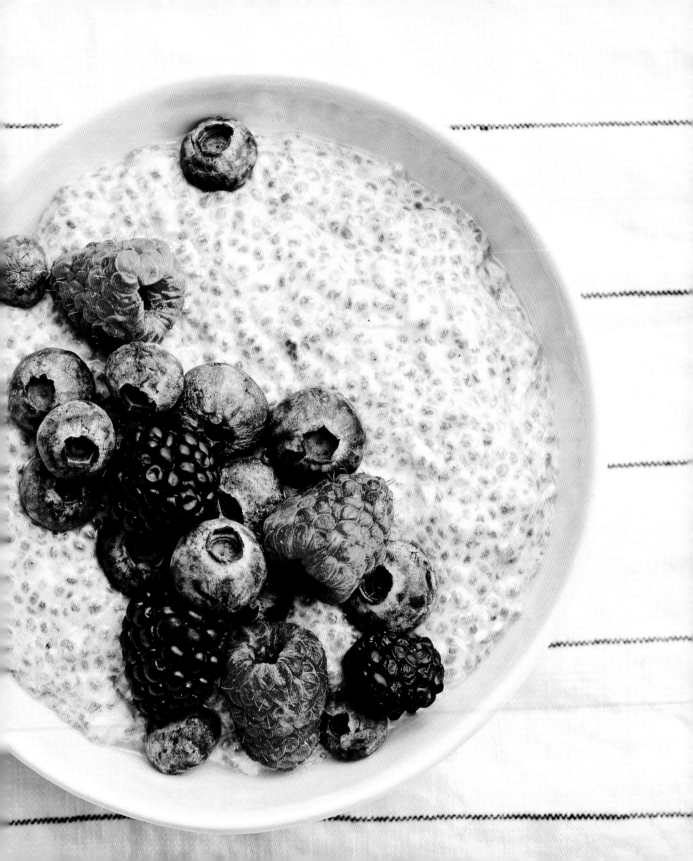

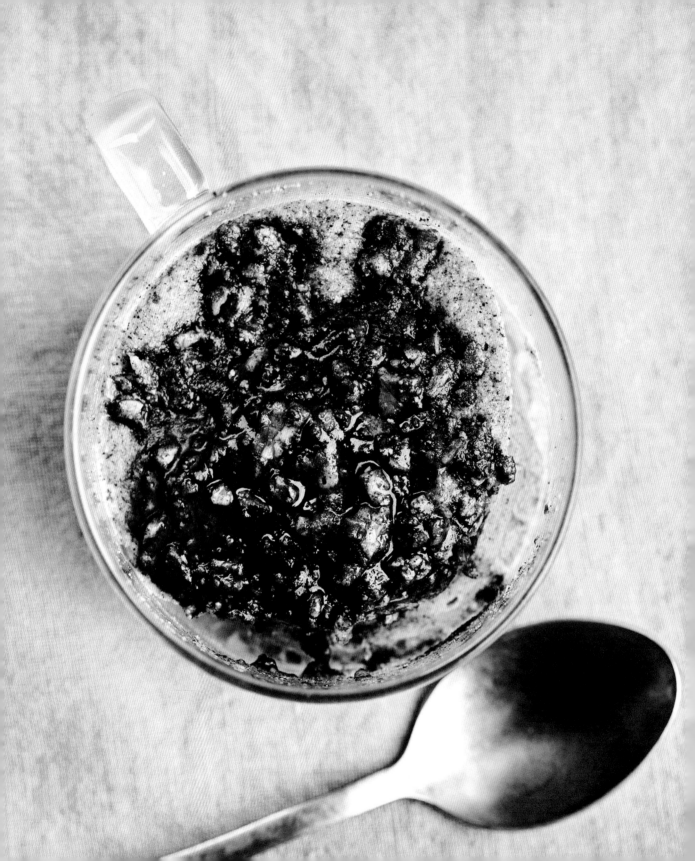

single-serving microwave coffee cake in a mug

Craving coffee cake without the hassle? Enter this single-serve mug cake! A blend of almond and coconut flour provides a high-fiber, high-protein base that's a lot better for blood sugars for this deliciously simple morning treat.

gluten-free | high fiber | high protein | quick & simple | yield: 1 mug cake

CAKE

½ tbsp (7 g) coconut oil, melted

2 tsp (10 ml) maple syrup

1 large egg (57 g)

2 tbsp (30 ml) plain nonfat Greek yogurt

½ tsp vanilla extract

½ tsp almond extract

2 tbsp (12 g) almond flour

1½ tbsp (11 g) coconut flour

¼ tsp baking powder

1 tsp cinnamon

CRUMB TOPPING

½ tbsp (3 g) almond flour

½ tsp maple syrup

½ tsp cinnamon

½ tbsp (8 ml) melted coconut oil

1½ tsp (7 g) crushed walnuts

To make the cake batter, in a large mug, whisk together the melted coconut oil, maple syrup, egg, Greek yogurt, vanilla extract, and almond extract. Then, add the almond flour, coconut flour, baking powder, and cinnamon to the mug and stir until well combined.

For the crumb topping, in a separate bowl, combine the almond flour, maple syrup, cinnamon, melted coconut oil, and crushed walnuts. Sprinkle the crumb topping on the batter in the mug.

Microwave uncovered for 75 seconds, or until an inserted toothpick comes out clean. Enjoy immediately.

> TIP: You can make the batter the night before and let it sit covered in the fridge overnight. In the morning, simply remove the cover and pop it in the microwave when you are ready for breakfast.

Nutrition Info (Serving size: 1 mug cake): Calories: 445, Total Fat: 32 g, Saturated Fat: 16 g, Total Carbohydrates: 27 g, Sugar: 13 g, Fiber: 8 g, Sodium: 224 mg, Protein: 15 g

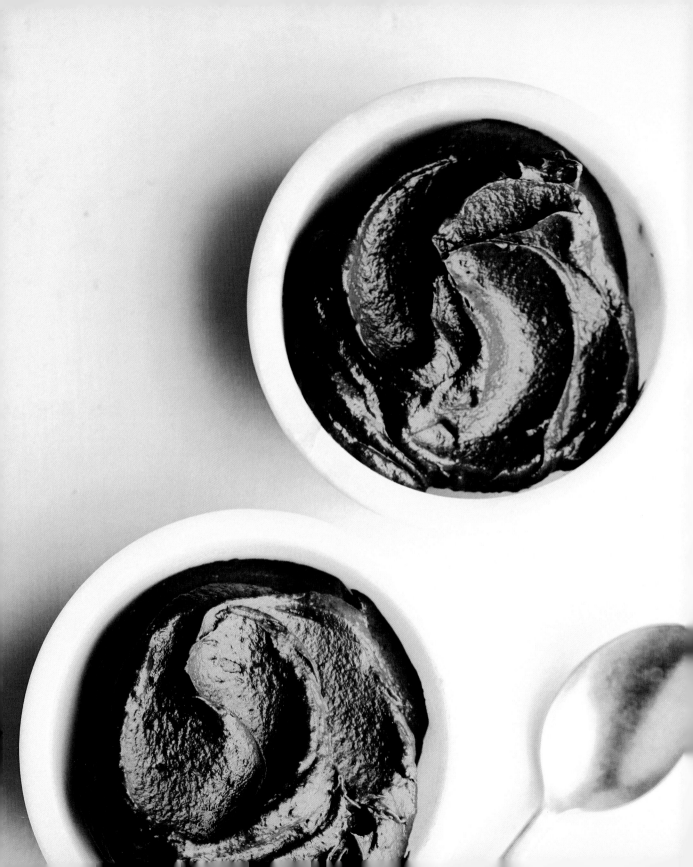

easy no-bake treats

Think of your common store-bought protein bars or energy bites. They're typically pretty pricey and can often be loaded with sugar. And unfortunately, they may not actually offer all that much protein or energy. But don't worry! It's actually quite easy to make these types of snacks and desserts at home . . . and with the no-bake treats in this chapter, we don't have to turn the oven on at all!

Having a good collection of recipes for easy no-bake treats can make balancing blood sugars a lot easier. These types of recipes are perfect for a quick morning or afternoon snack, and having quick and easy snack options to get you from one meal to the next is really helpful in maintaining consistent blood sugars. And feeling like we're enjoying a delicious dessert at the same time just makes it a win-win scenario!

You'll notice we use a lot of common ingredients in these no-bake recipes. By using a similar base recipe and then changing the flavor profiles, the recipe options are endless. Each of these ingredients helps balance our blood sugars, including:

- **Nuts:** Nuts give us a lot of that nutrient density we need, and are made of primarily fat and protein, which are essential in slowing down your body's blood sugar response.
- **Dried fruit:** Dried fruit and dates are a natural source of sweetness that also offer fiber and antioxidants. And when we puree or blend them up with nuts, we get a dough-like texture that is super easy to work with.
- **Oats and almond flour:** Oats and almond flour provide complex carbohydrates and act as binders and moisture absorbers. With no-bake desserts, we don't have to worry about the food chemistry that comes along with baked goods, so we can combine ingredients until we reach the consistency we like without needing to consider how they'll react in an oven.
- **Cooked beans and lentils:** Mashed up beans and lentils are fairly mild tasting and provide complex carbohydrates (fiber) and protein . . . perfect for making things like Chocolate Chip Pecan Edible Cookie Dough (page 109).

Whether you want to whip up some Cherry Pie Energy Balls (page 102), Better-for-You High-Protein Brownie Bites (page 110), or one of the other delicious treats in this chapter, you can be confident they'll have the fat, fiber, and protein you need to keep you energized throughout your day

cherry pie energy balls

These are the perfect little bites of sweetness for an afternoon pick-me-up or a pre-workout snack. Nuts provide wholesome fats while the unsweetened dried fruit, flax seeds, and oats give a dose of fiber to help balance your blood sugars. The result is a portable snack that's delicious and naturally sweet.

dairy-free | no added sugar | quick & simple | yield: 16 energy balls

½ cup (55 g) raw pecans

½ cup (73 g) raw cashews

½ cup (45 g) rolled oats

¾ cup (113 g) unsweetened dried cherries

2 Medjool dates, pitted

¼ cup (28 g) ground flax seeds

1 tsp cinnamon

This recipe couldn't be easier! In a high-power blender or food processor, simply add the pecans, cashews, oats, dried cherries, dates, flax seeds, and cinnamon and process on the highest setting until a cookie dough consistency forms. If needed, use 1 to 2 tablespoons (15 to 30 ml) of water or milk to help your blender or food processor along.

There's no need to refrigerate this dough; simply use a cookie scoop (or your hands) to create evenly sized energy balls.

Store your finished energy balls in the fridge for up to 2 weeks or the freezer for up to 3 months.

TIP: Be sure to use unsweetened dried cherries to keep the sugar in this recipe low. If you cannot find unsweetened dried cherries, feel free to substitute an equal amount of another unsweetened dried fruit of choice.

Nutrition Info (Serving size: 2 energy balls): Calories: 182, Total Fat: 10 g, Saturated Fat: 1 g, Total Carbohydrates: 21 g, Sugar: 11 g, Fiber: 4 g, Sodium: 2 mg, Protein: 4 g

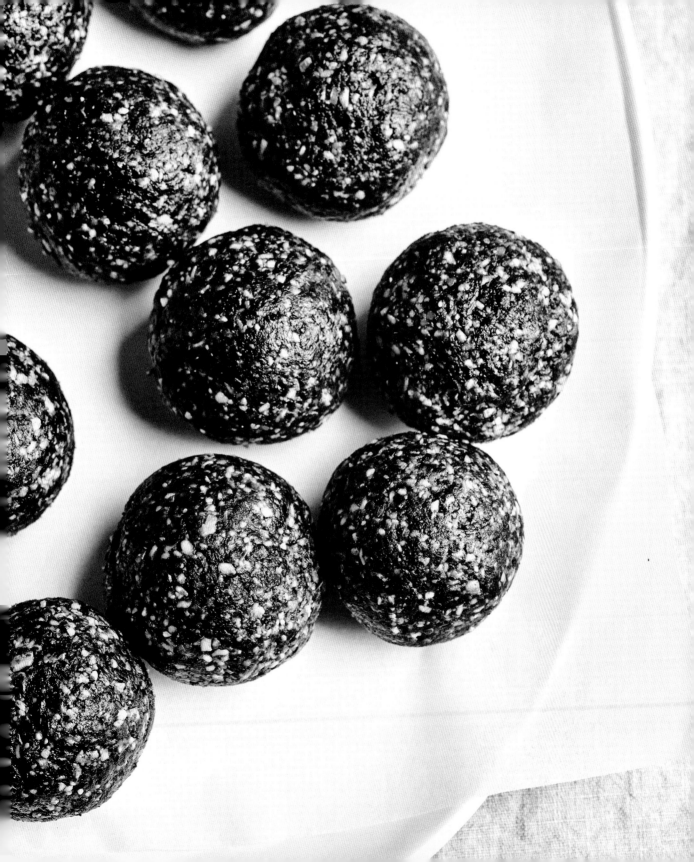

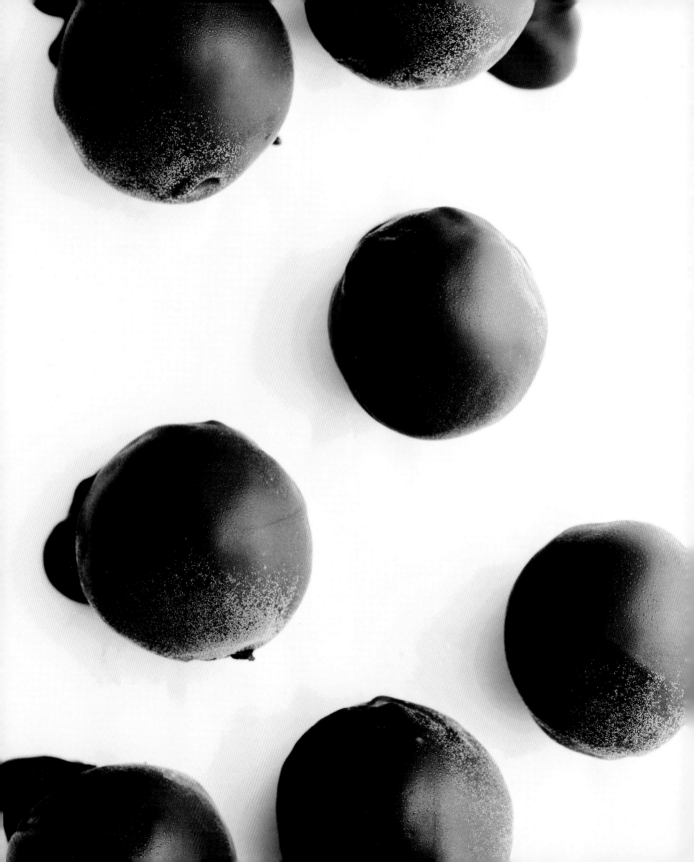

chocolate peppermint truffles

Nuts and dates are the stars of these truffles. When blended, these ingredients create a dreamy dough consistency that is naturally sweet and high in fiber, protein, and healthy fats. It's delicious alone, but the peppermint extract mixed in chocolate adds a fun and festive pop of flavor.

dairy-free | gluten-free | high fiber | high protein | yield: 12 truffles

8 Medjool dates, pitted

½ cup (59 g) walnuts

¼ cup (24 g) almond flour

4 tbsp (28 g) ground flax seeds

1 tsp cinnamon

1 tsp vanilla extract

⅓ cup (55 g) semi-sweet chocolate chips

¼ tsp peppermint extract

1 tbsp (14 g) coconut oil, melted

In a high-power blender or food processor, blend the dates, walnuts, almond flour, ground flax seeds, cinnamon, and vanilla extract until a dough-like consistency is reached, 30 to 45 seconds.

Use a cookie scoop to form 12 balls and set them aside.

Next, in a microwave-safe bowl, mix the chocolate chips, peppermint extract, and melted coconut oil. Heat the mixture in the microwave until liquid and smooth, 45 to 60 seconds. Dip each ball into the melted chocolate mixture until coated. Add them to a parchment-lined baking sheet and put them in the freezer to set for at least 3 hours.

Store in the refrigerator for up to 2 weeks, or in the freezer for up to 2 months.

TIP: Using a fork to spin the truffle around in the chocolate can help coat it in a thin, even layer.

Nutrition Info (Serving size: 2 truffles): Calories: 257, Total Fat: 15 g, Saturated Fat: 4 g, Total Carbohydrates: 30 g, Sugar: 22 g, Fiber: 5 g, Sodium: 1 mg, Protein: 5 g

oatmeal cookie protein bites

The humble cannellini bean gets a major upgrade in this recipe. It's the perfect addition because of its mild taste and creamy consistency when blended . . . not to mention cannellini beans' impressive nutrient profile of fiber, protein, and iron. Vanilla and almond extract provide that classic oatmeal cookie taste and alleviate the need to add excessive amounts of sweetener.

dairy-free | yield: 24 bites

1 (15-oz [425-g]) can cannellini beans, rinsed and drained

¼ cup (65 g) cashew butter

½ cup (51 g) almond flour

1 cup (90 g) rolled oats, divided

⅓ cup (80 ml) maple syrup

2 tsp (10 ml) vanilla extract

2 tsp (10 ml) almond extract

1 tbsp (8 g) cinnamon

In a high-power blender or food processor, combine the cannellini beans, cashew butter, almond flour, ½ cup (45 g) of oats, maple syrup, vanilla extract, almond extract, and cinnamon. Blend on the highest setting until smooth.

Then, fold in the other ½ cup (45 g) of oats to provide a more solid texture.

Next, using a cookie scoop, make 24 evenly sized bites. Freeze for at least 2 hours to set and enjoy!

You can store your protein bites in the refrigerator or the freezer. Store them in the refrigerator for up to 2 weeks, or in the freezer for up to 2 months.

TIP: You can find cashew butter near the almond and peanut butter in your grocery store. Feel free to substitute peanut butter or almond butter, but cashew butter gives a more "cookie dough" taste.

Nutrition Info (Serving size: 1 bite): Calories: 73, Total Fat: 3 g, Saturated Fat: 0 g, Total Carbohydrates: 10 g, Sugar: 3 g, Fiber: 2 g, Sodium: 51 mg, Protein: 2 g

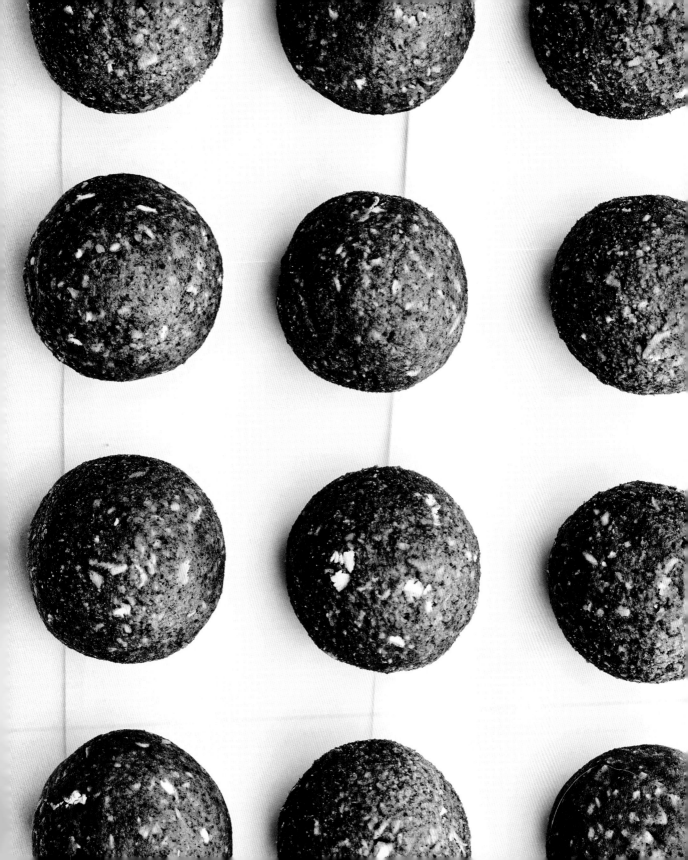

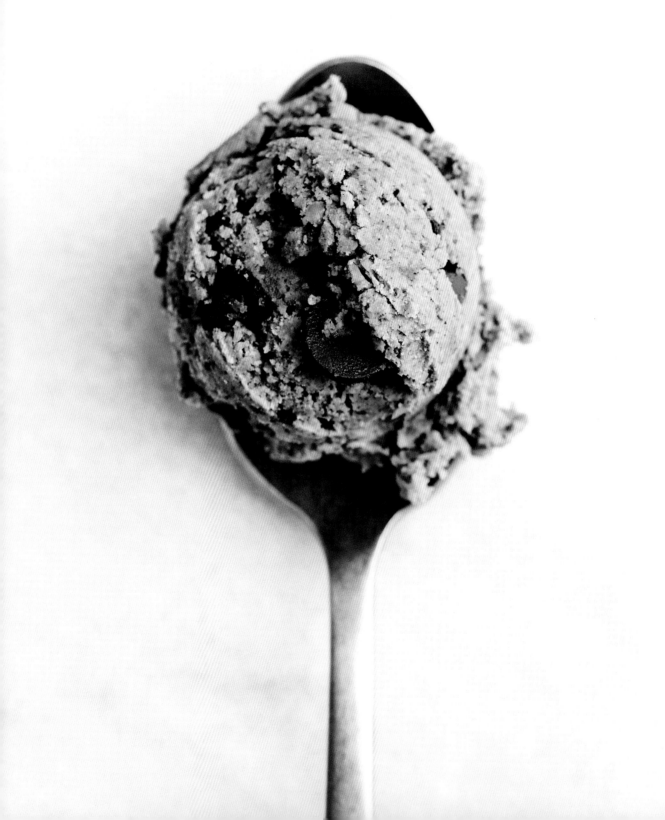

chocolate chip pecan edible cookie dough

Everyone knows cookie dough is the best part of baking! This one is designed for eating, not baking, though, and boasts a secret ingredient that gives it a unique protein and fiber boost—beans! And don't worry, you'll be so amazed at how delicious this cookie dough tastes, you'll never even know they're in there!

dairy-free | quick & simple | yield: 12 servings

1 (15-oz [425-g]) can cannellini beans, drained and rinsed

1 cup (109 g) raw pecans

¼ cup (30 g) coconut flour

¼ cup (23 g) rolled oats

1 tsp cinnamon

3 Medjool dates, pitted

1½ tbsp (23 ml) maple syrup

2 tsp (10 ml) vanilla extract

1 tsp almond extract

½ cup (84 g) semi-sweet chocolate chips

In a high-power blender or food processor, add the drained cannellini beans, pecans, coconut flour, oats, cinnamon, dates, maple syrup, vanilla extract, and almond extract. Blend on high until smooth, 20 to 30 seconds. If your mixture seems dry, add 1 to 2 tablespoons (15 to 30 ml) of water to the mixture until a dough-like consistency forms.

Carefully transfer the dough to a storage container or bowl and fold in the chocolate chips and enjoy!

You can keep your dough as is or roll it into balls if you prefer!

Store your cookie dough in the fridge in an airtight container for 3 to 4 days.

TIPS: Feel free to get creative and substitute ½ cup (75 g) of your favorite cookie mix-in for the chocolate chips.

Navy beans are a nice substitute for cannellini beans, as both are very mild tasting.

Nutrition Info (Serving size: about ¼ cup [60 g]): Calories: 162, Total Fat: 9 g, Saturated Fat: 2 g, Total Carbohydrates: 20 g, Sugar: 9 g, Fiber: 4 g, Sodium: 105 mg, Protein: 3 g

better-for-you high-protein brownie bites

Peanuts, peanut flour, and hemp seeds help give these bites a healthy dose of protein and blood sugar–friendly fats. And dates provide natural sweetness and fiber while serving as a binder for the remaining ingredients. You'll want to make these brownie bites over and over again!

dairy-free | gluten-free | high fiber | high protein | no added sugar | yield: 22 bites

¼ cup (30 g) coconut flour

1 cup (146 g) peanuts, shelled

¼ cup (28 g) ground flax seeds

¼ cup (30 g) peanut flour

¼ cup (22 g) unsweetened cocoa powder

10 Medjool dates, pitted

3 tbsp (30 g) hemp seeds

1 tbsp (14 g) coconut oil, melted

1 tsp vanilla extract

¼–½ cup (60–120 ml) unsweetened almond milk (as needed to blend)

To a high-power blender or food processor, add your coconut flour, peanuts, ground flax seeds, peanut flour, cocoa powder, dates, hemp seeds, coconut oil, vanilla extract, and ¼ cup (60 ml) of almond milk. Blend the ingredients together until a smooth cookie dough consistency forms, adding some of the additional almond milk as needed.

Carefully remove the dough from the food processor and transfer it to a bowl. Using a cookie scoop, form 22 bites. Freeze for at least 3 hours before enjoying them.

Store your brownie bites in the refrigerator for up to 2 weeks or in the freezer for up to 3 months.

TIPS: Use the second half of the almond milk as needed. You may need to adjust the quantity you use depending on the power of your blender and the stickiness of your dates.

You can typically find peanut flour, sometimes called powdered peanut butter, either in the baking aisle or with the other peanut butter jars in your local grocery store.

Nutrition Info (Serving size: 2 bites): Calories: 193, Total Fat: 11 g, Saturated Fat: 3 g, Total Carbohydrates: 20 g, Sugar: 12 g, Fiber: 5 g, Sodium: 33 mg, Protein: 7 g

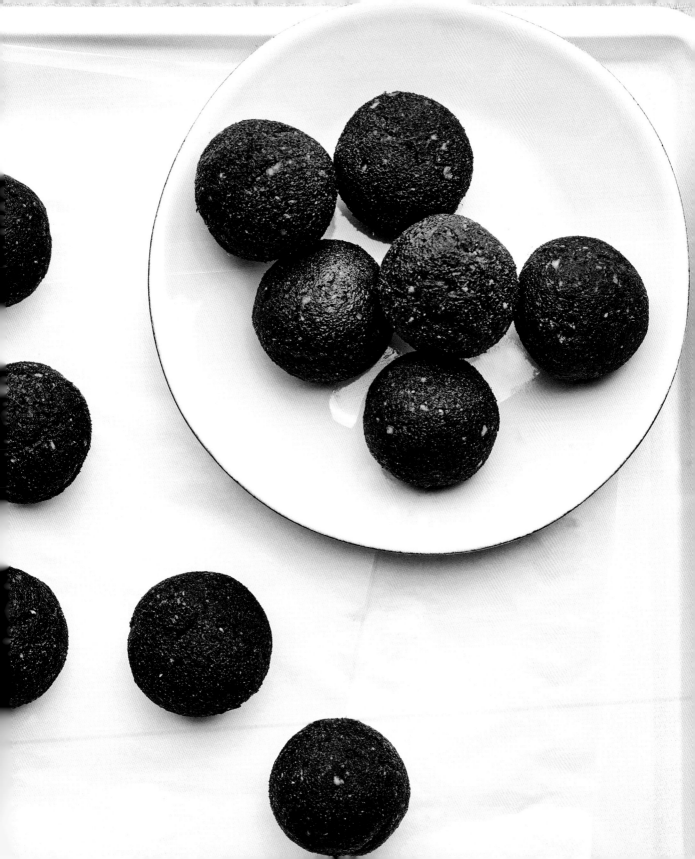

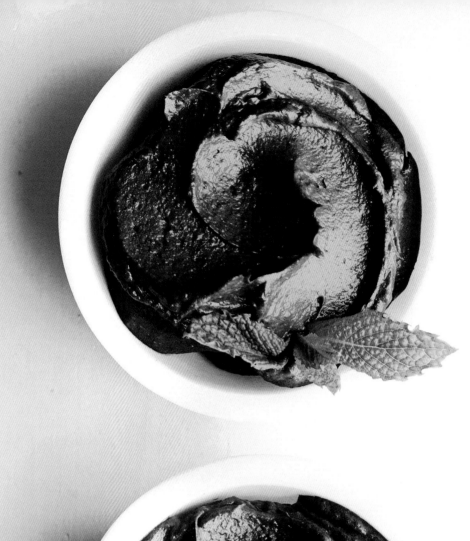
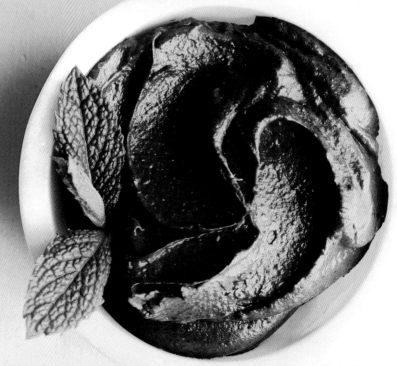

easy chocolate fudge avocado mousse

Avocado provides a creamy, high-fiber base for this decadent-tasting mousse! It's delicious, blood sugar friendly, and totally satisfying. The rich dark chocolate flavor combined with all those blood sugar–balancing avocado fats are the perfect way to satisfy your sweet tooth!

dairy-free | gluten-free | high fiber | no added sugar | yield: 6 servings

2 medium avocados, peeled and pit removed, cubed

4 Medjool dates, pitted

½ cup (120 ml) unsweetened almond milk

2 tbsp (20 g) chia seeds

2 tbsp (11 g) unsweetened cocoa powder

2 tsp (10 ml) vanilla extract

To a blender or food processor, add your avocado, dates, almond milk, chia seeds, cocoa powder, and vanilla extract. Blend on high until smooth and creamy, about 30 seconds. Chill the mousse for 2 hours before serving.

Store your chocolate mousse in a sealed container in the fridge for up to 2 days.

TIP: Chill your chocolate mousse for at least 2 hours before serving, or you can use frozen cubed avocado when you make the mousse and enjoy it right away.

Nutrition Info (Serving size: about ⅓ cup [80 g]): Calories: 155, Total Fat: 9 g, Saturated Fat: 1 g, Total Carbohydrates: 19 g, Sugar: 11 g, Fiber: 7 g, Sodium: 17 mg, Protein: 3 g

almond butter & raspberry jelly bars

The classic PB&J gets a dessert makeover in this simple recipe. Oats, almond butter, and flax provide a high-fiber base with plenty of healthy fats. Dates and freeze-dried raspberries provide natural sweetness and an extra punch of fiber.

dairy-free | high fiber | high protein | no added sugar | yield: 8 bars

¾ cup (194 g) unsweetened almond butter

¾ cup (68 g) rolled oats

⅓ cup (37 g) ground flax seeds

1⅛ cup (23 g) freeze-dried raspberries

5 Medjool dates, pitted

1 tbsp (15 ml) vanilla extract

2 tbsp (30 ml) unsweetened almond milk

In a high-power blender or food processor, combine the almond butter, rolled oats, flax seeds, freeze-dried raspberries, dates, vanilla extract, and almond milk. Blend until a cookie dough consistency forms.

Using a rubber spatula, add the dough to a parchment-lined 8 x 8–inch (20 x 20–cm) square pan. Cut the dough into eight bars, and place the pan in the freezer for at least 2 hours before enjoying. You should be able to separate the bars easily when you remove them from the freezer. If not, allow them to thaw for about 10 minutes and they'll come apart very easily!

Store your bars in the freezer in a sealed container for up to 3 months.

> TIP: Freeze-dried fruit is typically found with the dried fruit and nuts in the grocery store. Feel free to experiment with an equal amount of your favorite variety of freeze-dried fruit.

Nutrition Info (Serving size: 1 bar): Calories: 248, Total Fat: 15 g, Saturated Fat: 1 g, Total Carbohydrates: 23 g, Sugar: 9 g, Fiber: 6 g, Sodium: 5 mg, Protein: 8 g

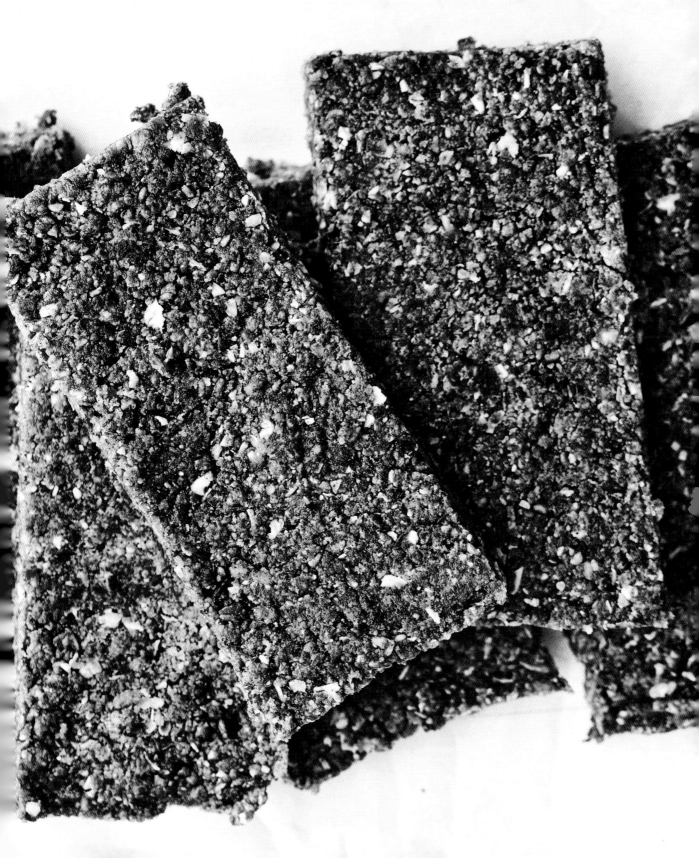

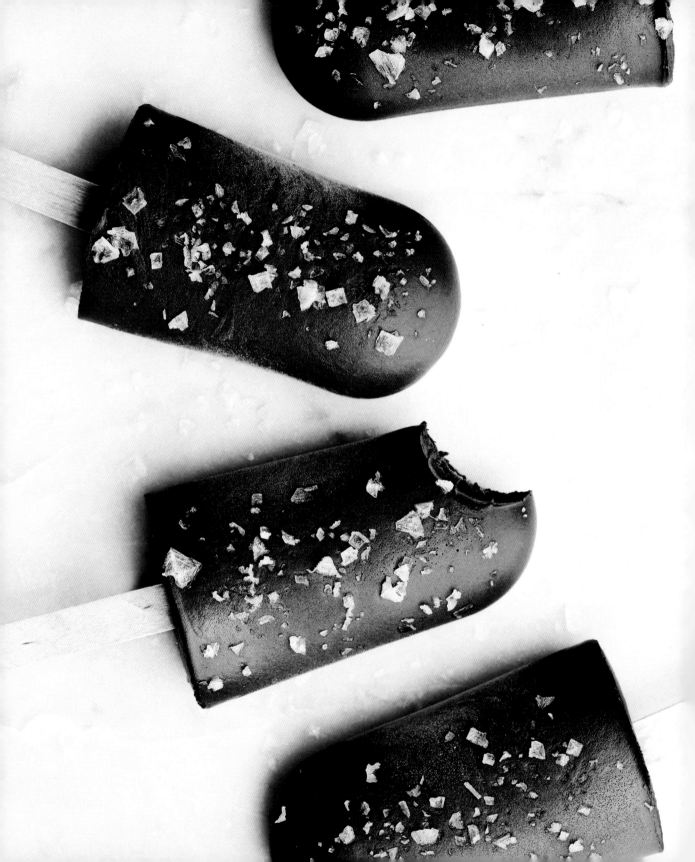

fantastically frozen desserts

Whether it's popsicles or ice cream, freezer fudge or milkshakes, frozen desserts often come with a hefty dose of sugar and saturated fat. In fact, some restaurant versions of our favorite frozen classics can top over 50 grams of sugar! Crazy, right?

Well, don't worry. You know I've got you covered with these just-as-delicious, and more nutritious, homemade options. When we're in our own kitchen, we can rely on other types of ingredients that don't actually add sugar to sweeten these frozen desserts up, like:

- **Extracts:** Vanilla, almond, and peppermint extracts are perfect for adding a huge punch of flavor and sweetness without adding sugar.
- **Lemon zest:** Lemon zest adds such a delicious, fragrantly sweet taste to our Strawberry Lemonade Ice Pops (page 121).
- **Salt:** Believe it or not, adding salt to a dish can actually enhance naturally occurring sweet flavors to make them taste even sweeter. Don't believe me? Just give the Dark Chocolate Sea Salt Fudge Pops (page 129) a try!

Many of these recipes are also a great way to get young kids in the kitchen for mixing and stirring, for treats the whole family can enjoy!

healthy mint chocolate chip ice cream in a jar

This is a healthy ice cream you can make in your blender. Frozen bananas provide natural sweetness and a creamy ice cream–like texture. Hemp seeds are tasteless, nutrient-packed blood sugar–balancing powerhouses filled with protein, beneficial fats, and iron. You can serve these in cute jars for perfect portions and a fun presentation!

dairy-free | gluten-free | high protein | quick & simple | yield: 4 servings

2 bananas, chopped and frozen

4 tbsp (40 g) hemp seeds

1 cup (30 g) baby spinach

¼ tsp peppermint extract

½ cup (120 ml) unsweetened almond milk

¼ cup (42 g) semi-sweet chocolate chips

Whipped cream for topping (optional)

Shaved chocolate for topping (optional)

In a high-power blender or food processor, blend your bananas, hemp seeds, baby spinach, peppermint extract, and almond milk on high for 30 to 45 seconds.

Next, add the chocolate chips to the mixture and blend on low for 5 to 10 seconds to lightly incorporate.

Serve your ice cream in mason jars. And if you want to get extra fancy, you can top it with whipped cream and a sprinkle of additional chocolate.

Enjoy your ice cream immediately or store it in a loaf pan in the freezer for up to 1 month. If you store it in the freezer, let it sit at room temperature for 30 minutes before serving and use an ice cream scooper to serve.

TIPS: Frozen bananas give this ice cream its creamy texture; don't skip this step!

Hemp seeds can be found in the supplement section of your grocery store near chia seeds, flax seeds, and protein powder.

Nutrition Info (Serving size: ¼ of the recipe, about ½ cup [120 g]): Calories: 164, Total Fat: 9 g, Saturated Fat: 2 g, Total Carbohydrates: 21 g, Sugar: 13 g, Fiber: 3 g, Sodium: 28 mg, Protein: 5 g

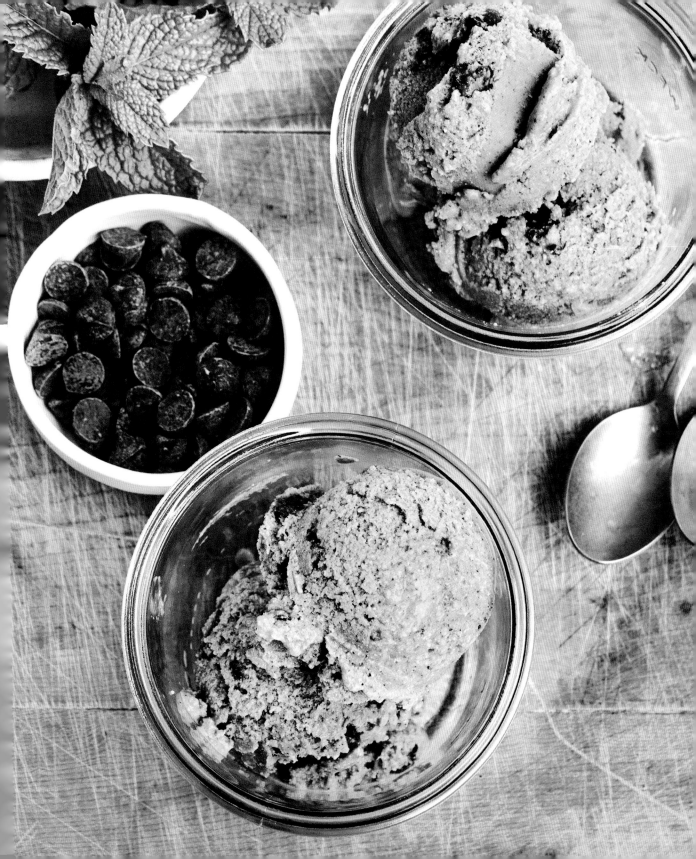

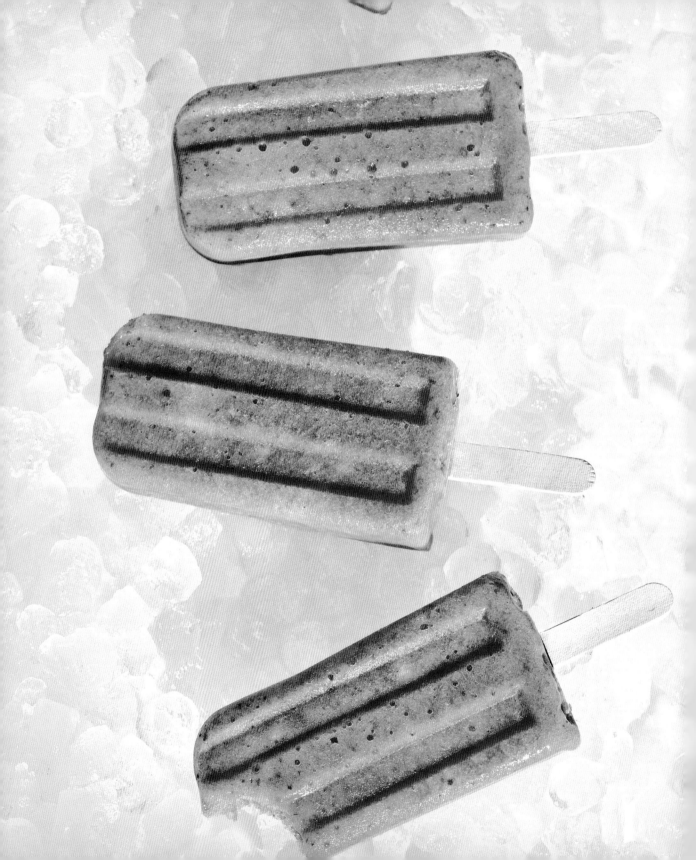

strawberry lemonade ice pops

These tart and sweet refreshing treats are perfect for a hot summer day. Strawberries provide a touch of natural sweetness and fiber while collagen adds a protein boost that won't alter the flavor or texture of the popsicles.

dairy-free | gluten-free | yield: 4 ice pops

2 cups (288 g) frozen strawberries

½ cup (120 ml) lemon juice

1 tbsp (6 g) lemon zest

½ cup (120 ml) water

¼ cup (28 g) collagen powder

2 tsp (10 ml) honey

In a high-power blender, blend your frozen strawberries, lemon juice, lemon zest, water, collagen, and honey on high speed.

Pour the mixture into four popsicle molds and freeze until solid. Make sure to let them freeze for at least 4 hours before enjoying.

Store the ice pops in the freezer for up to 1 month.

TIP: The collagen powder can be found near the supplements in your grocery store or at your local drug store.

Nutrition Info (Serving size: 1 ice pop): Calories: 60, Total Fat: 0 g, Saturated Fat: 0 g, Total Carbohydrates: 11 g, Sugar: 7 g, Fiber: 2 g, Sodium: 12 mg, Protein: 4 g

frozen yogurt blueberry bites

These creamy, tart but sweet bites are the perfect antidote to a hot day. Lemon pairs beautifully with blueberries, which are naturally sweet and filled with fiber and antioxidants that give these bites their distinct deep purple hue. Walnuts add a crunch and boost of omega-3 fatty acids, which helps to reduce inflammation and promote stable blood sugars.

gluten-free | high protein | yield: 12 bites

5 oz (140 ml) plain low-fat Greek yogurt

2 tbsp (30 ml) honey

1 tsp lemon juice

½ tsp lemon zest

⅓ cup (39 g) crushed walnuts

1 cup (148 g) blueberries, fresh or frozen

In a bowl, whisk the yogurt, honey, lemon juice, and lemon zest until smooth. Then fold in the crushed walnuts and blueberries. Pour the mixture into an ice cube tray and freeze until solid, at least 2 hours, before enjoying.

Store in the freezer for up to 3 months.

TIP: If they are too hard to bite into, let them sit for 15 to 20 minutes before enjoying.

Nutrition Info (Serving size: 3 bites): Calories: 143, Total Fat: 7 g, Saturated Fat: 1 g, Total Carbohydrates: 17 g, Sugar: 14 g, Fiber: 2 g, Sodium: 13 mg, Protein: 5 g

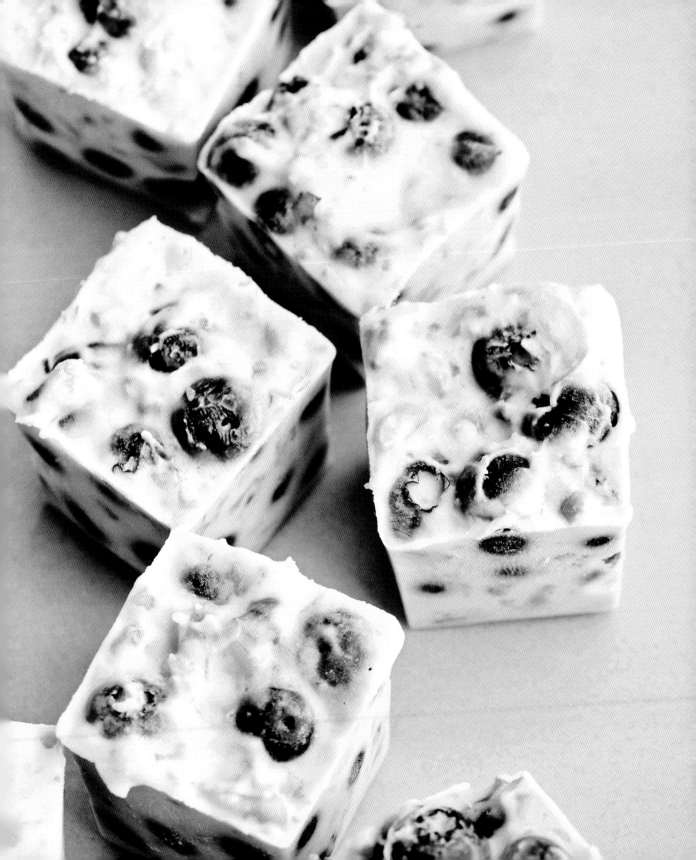

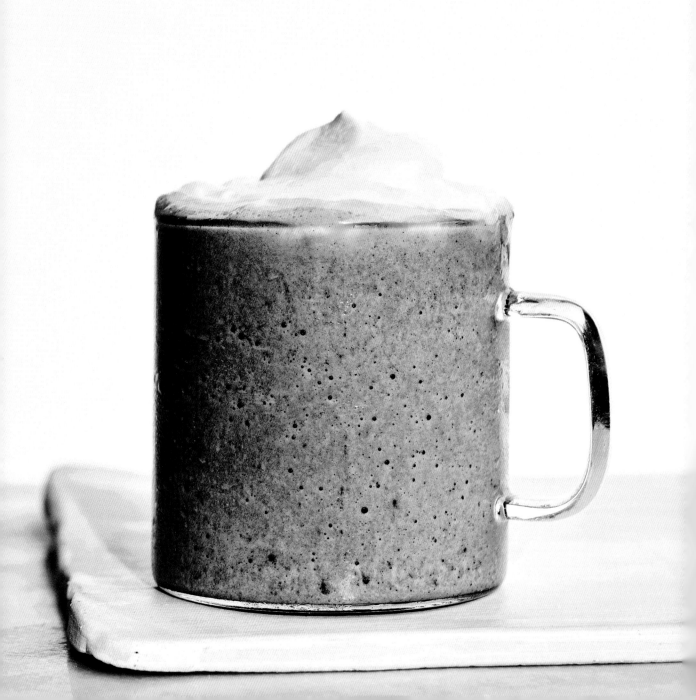

cinnamon frozen hot chocolate

Cinnamon frozen hot chocolate is a delicious oxymoron! This drink (it has an almost smoothie-like consistency) is naturally sweetened with banana and adds a hefty dose of protein from collagen powder. It's also high in fiber from banana and cocoa powder. All that protein and fiber make for the perfect blood sugar–friendly frozen dessert!

dairy-free | gluten-free | high fiber | high protein | quick & simple | yield: 1 serving

½ cup (120 ml) almond milk, frozen into ice cubes

1 cup (240 ml) almond milk

1 banana, chopped and frozen

3 tbsp (20 g) collagen powder

2 tsp (4 g) unsweetened cocoa powder

1 tsp cinnamon

2 tbsp (5 g) whipped cream

In a high-power blender, add the frozen almond milk cubes, almond milk, frozen banana chunks, collagen, cocoa powder, and cinnamon. Blend on high until smooth, 30 to 45 seconds.

Pour your frozen hot chocolate into your preferred cup, top with the whipped cream, and enjoy immediately.

TIPS: Frozen almond milk and banana give this drink a smoothie-like consistency, but the flavor is still there if you don't have time to freeze them ahead of time.

If you cannot find collagen, an equal amount of chocolate protein powder would also work, but I recommend reducing the added cocoa powder to 1 teaspoon.

Nutrition Info (Serving size: 1 recipe): Calories: 235, Total Fat: 4 g, Saturated Fat: 1 g, Total Carbohydrates: 34 g, Sugar: 16 g, Fiber: 7 g, Sodium: 205 mg, Protein: 21 g

peanut butter chocolate freezer fudge

Peanut butter is fantastic straight from the jar, so you don't need many more ingredients to create a satisfying fudge. It's also high in protein and healthy fats, which is an added bonus when using it as the base of a dessert. Vanilla extract, sea salt, and chocolate chips add extra flair without a lot of added sugar to make this freezer fudge your new favorite treat!

dairy-free | gluten-free | yield: 20 pieces

½ cup (129 g) smooth-style unsweetened peanut butter

2 tbsp (27 g) coconut oil, melted

½ tsp vanilla extract

¼ tsp sea salt

¼ cup (42 g) semi-sweet chocolate chips

In a large mixing bowl, whisk together the peanut butter, coconut oil, vanilla extract, and sea salt.

Pour the mixture into an ice cube tray, filling each cube only about halfway. Set the tray aside.

Next, melt the chocolate chips in 30 second increments in the microwave or using a double boiler for 3 to 4 minutes. Spoon the melted chocolate on top of the peanut butter mixture in the ice cube trays.

Freeze for at least 2 hours and enjoy.

Keep the fudge in the freezer for up to 3 months.

TIP: Salted or unsalted peanut butter will work in this recipe.

Nutrition Info (Serving size: 2 pieces): Calories: 122, Total Fat: 11 g, Saturated Fat: 4 g, Total Carbohydrates: 6 g, Sugar: 4 g, Fiber: 3 g, Sodium: 63 mg, Protein: 3 g

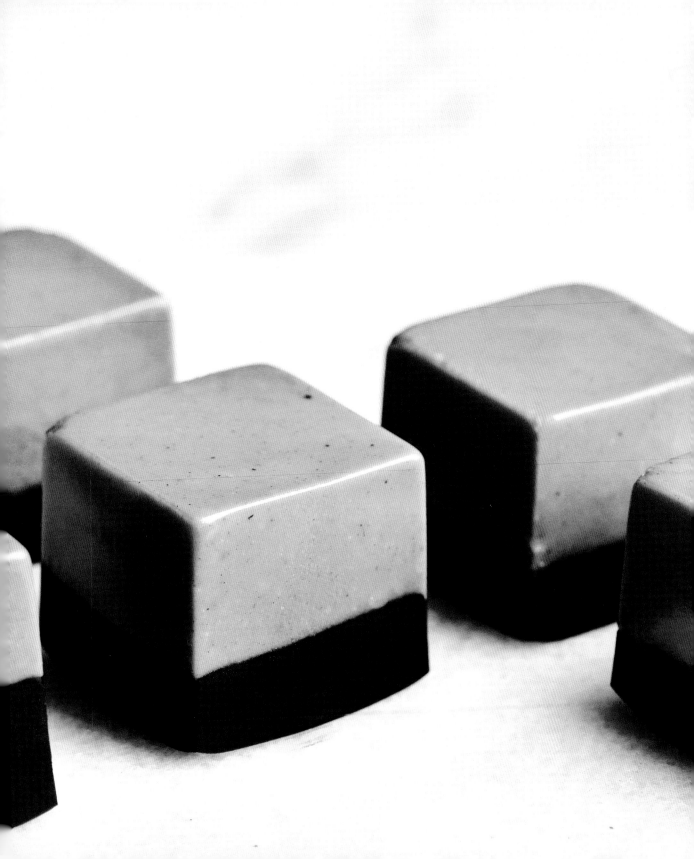

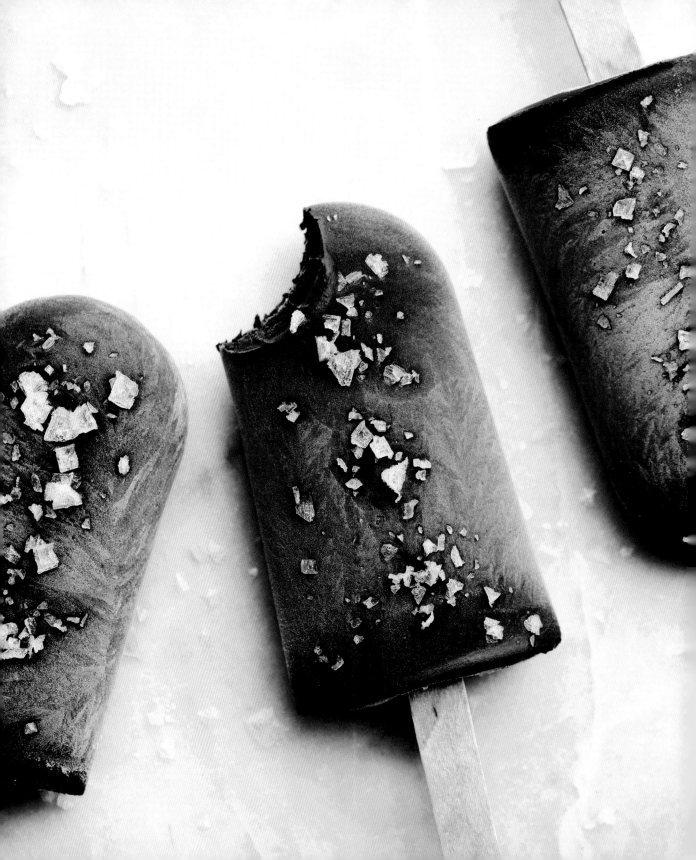

dark chocolate sea salt fudge pops

Nothing quite hits the spot like a delicious homemade fudge pop. For this recipe, we've added in some Greek yogurt and almond butter to increase both the fat content and protein! Both of these nutrients help to promote stable blood sugars.

gluten-free | high protein | yield: 8 fudge pops

8 oz (240 ml) half & half cream

1 cup (240 ml) plain 2% Greek yogurt

2 tbsp (30 g) unsweetened almond butter

1 tsp vanilla extract

¼ cup (60 ml) maple syrup

¼ cup (22 g) unsweetened cocoa powder

¼ cup (42 g) semi-sweet chocolate chips

½ tsp flaked sea salt, plus more to sprinkle on top

In a medium-sized pot, whisk together the half & half, Greek yogurt, almond butter, vanilla extract, maple syrup, and cocoa powder until fully combined into one uniform mixture. It should resemble creamy chocolate milk.

Place the pot on the stove over low heat. Add the chocolate chips and sea salt to the pot and stir constantly with a small whisk or rubber spatula until the chocolate chips are fully melted.

Pour the mixture into your popsicle molds and freeze for 4 to 6 hours, or until frozen solid. Remove the fudge pops from the mold when you are ready to eat one and sprinkle with a bit of the flaked sea salt (just a small amount goes a long way!).

Fudge pops will keep in the freezer for up to 3 months.

TIPS: If you don't have half & half on hand, use any type of milk you prefer.

I prefer the creaminess of 2% Greek yogurt, but you can also use any type of yogurt you like.

You can adjust the sweetness level of these fudge pops by changing the amount of maple syrup. Use more or less if you'd like! Just remember, any substitutions will change the nutrition facts below.

Nutrition Info (Serving size: 1 fudge pop): Calories: 153, Total Fat: 9 g, Saturated Fat: 4 g, Total Carbohydrates: 16 g, Sugar: 11 g, Fiber: 2 g, Sodium: 169 mg, Protein: 5 g

mango cream sorbet

This is a creamy, perfectly sweet sorbet that you can make in your blender. Sweet mango and coconut milk are swirled together for the perfect flavor combo. And chia and hemp seeds are seamlessly blended in for a fiber and protein boost to keep blood sugars stable.

dairy-free | gluten-free | high protein | no added sugar | quick & simple | yield: 4 servings

¾ cup (180 ml) canned coconut milk

2 cups (280 g) frozen mango chunks

2 tbsp (20 g) chia seeds

3 tbsp (30 g) hemp seeds

To a blender, add the coconut milk, mango, chia seeds, and hemp seeds and blend on the highest setting for about 30 seconds to create a creamy sorbet.

Enjoy immediately or freeze in a loaf pan for up to 2 months. If frozen, let it sit at room temperature for about 20 minutes before using an ice cream scooper to serve.

TIPS: You may need to use a tamper to keep things moving in your blender. If your blender doesn't have this tool, adding ¼ to ½ cup (60 to 120 ml) of water will help also! (Add about ¼ cup [60 ml] of water at a time.)

Freeze ¼ cup (60 ml) or more of the coconut milk in ice cube trays to create an even thicker sorbet consistency.

Nutrition Info (Serving size: about ½ cup [120 g]): Calories: 201, Total Fat: 14 g, Saturated Fat: 8 g, Total Carbohydrates: 17 g, Sugar: 12 g, Fiber: 3 g, Sodium: 13 mg, Protein: 5 g

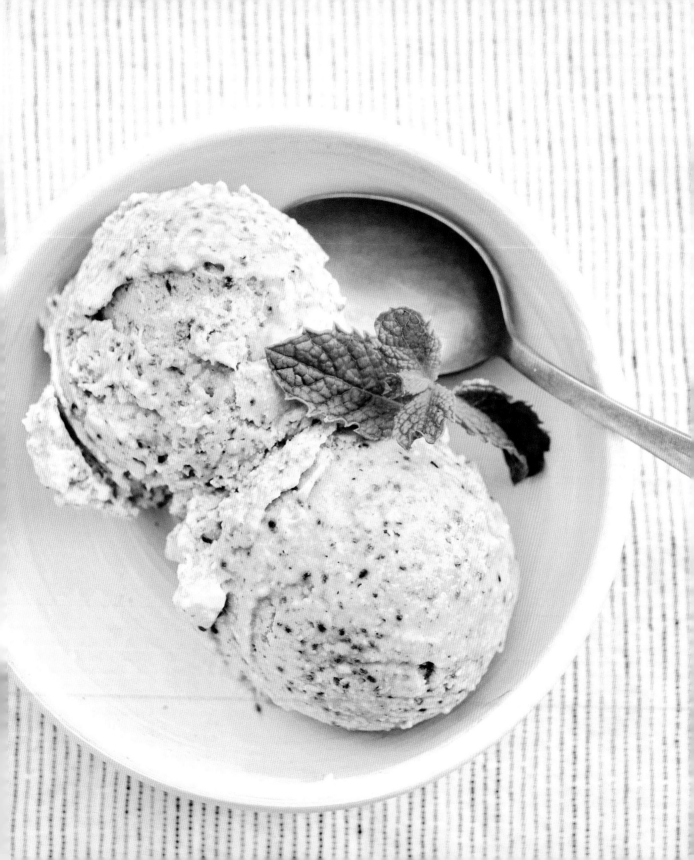

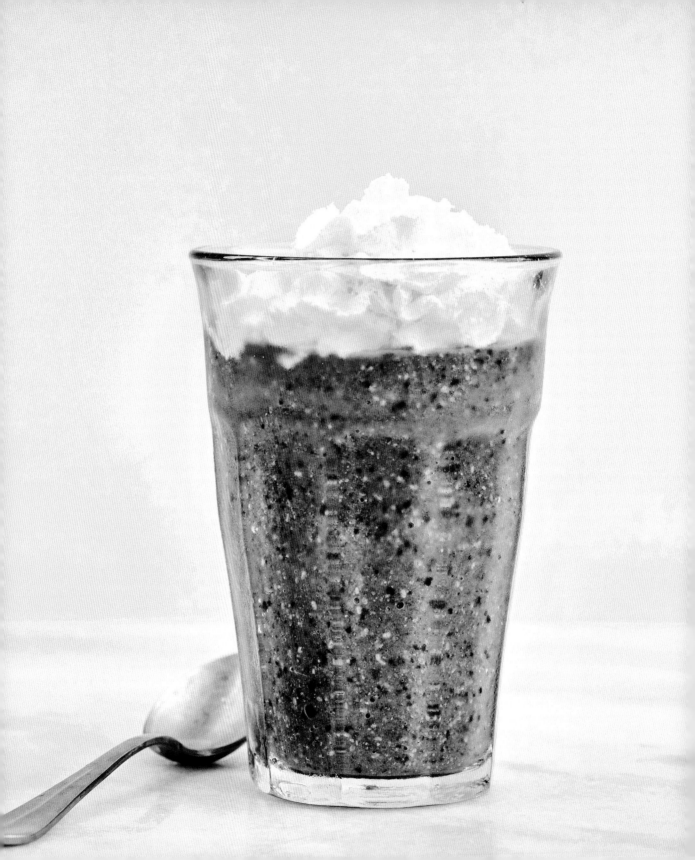

cherry vanilla milkshake

Frozen fruit and chia seeds create a naturally sweet treat that is high in fiber. This milkshake will make you think you've taken a detour to the ice cream shop—it's that good! And a dollop of whipped cream on top is added to enhance the sweetness without adding a ton of sugar.

gluten-free | quick & simple | high fiber | high protein | yield: 1 serving

¾ cup (116 g) frozen cherries

2 tbsp (20 g) chia seeds

½ cup (120 ml) unsweetened almond milk

2 tsp (10 ml) vanilla extract

2 tbsp (6 g) whipped cream, optional

To a high-power blender, add the frozen cherries, chia seeds, almond milk, and vanilla extract and blend on the highest setting until smooth, 20 to 30 seconds. Top with the whipped cream.

Enjoy immediately.

> TIP: Frozen fruit makes this treat even creamier, but fresh fruit will work also.

Nutrition Info (Serving size: 1 milkshake): Calories: 227, Total Fat: 11 g, Saturated Fat: 1 g, Total Carbohydrates: 26 g, Sugar: 13 g, Fiber: 8 g, Sodium: 82 mg, Protein: 6 g

frozen yogurt blackberry mint bark

Greek yogurt creates a tangy, high-protein blank canvas for this frozen treat. Blackberries, pistachios, and fresh mint are added for fiber, fat, and flavor. And a drizzle of honey adds just enough sweetness to make this a blood sugar–friendly dessert.

gluten-free | high protein | yield: 4 servings

5 oz (140 ml) plain low-fat, unsweetened Greek yogurt

2 tbsp (30 ml) honey

¾ cup (108 g) blackberries

¼ cup (25 g) shelled pistachios, chopped

1 tbsp (6 g) chopped fresh mint leaves

Line a baking sheet with parchment paper and set aside.

In a medium-sized bowl, whisk together the yogurt and honey until smooth. Lightly mash the blackberries with the back of a spoon and fold them into the yogurt mixture. Then spread the mixture onto the parchment-lined baking sheet. Sprinkle the pistachios and mint leaves on top. Freeze until solid, at least 2 hours. Break into four pieces and serve.

Keep in the freezer for 2 to 3 months.

> TIP: This recipe would work well with an equal amount of raspberries, blueberries, or strawberries. You could also substitute an equal amount of walnuts or pecans in place of the pistachios.

Nutrition Info (Serving size: 1 piece): Calories: 112, Total Fat: 4 g, Saturated Fat: 1 g, Total Carbohydrates: 15 g, Sugar: 12 g, Fiber: 2 g, Sodium: 13 mg, Protein: 6 g

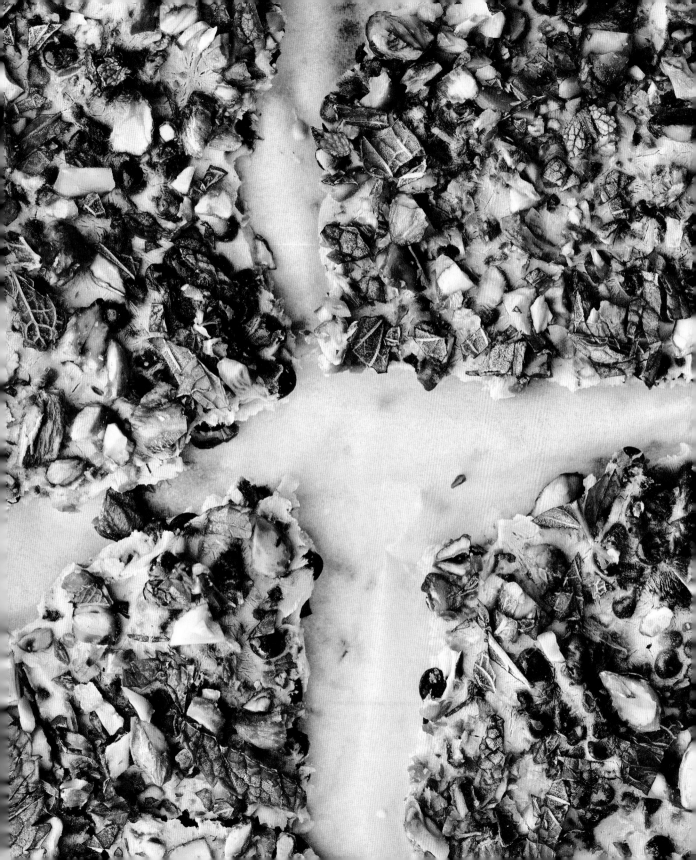

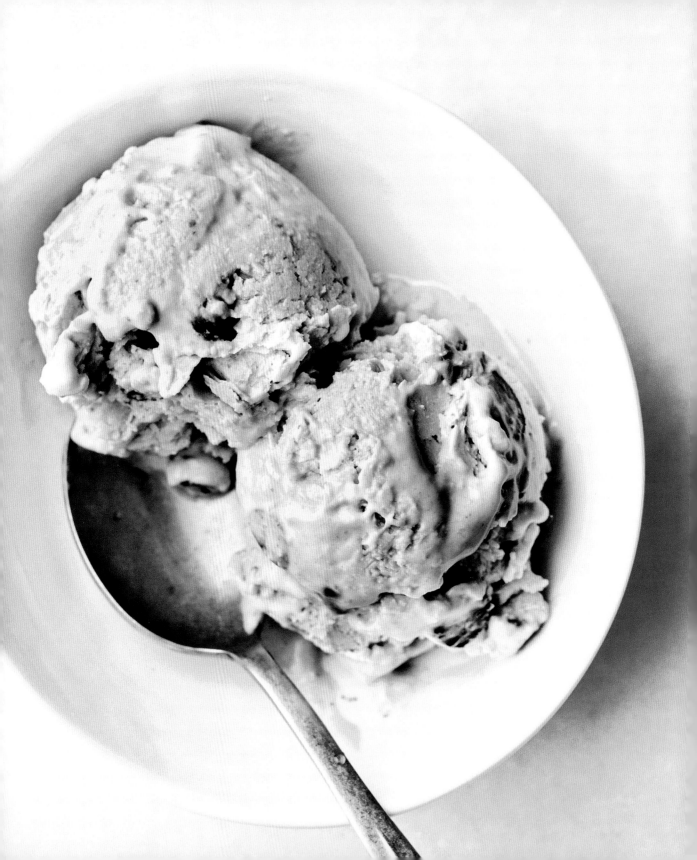

peanut butter chocolate chip "frozen yogurt"

Making frozen yogurt at home using Greek yogurt is an easy way to make this a high-protein, more blood sugar–friendly dessert. Using both peanut butter and peanut flour gives this fro-yo an incredible texture and bold taste with a boost of healthy fats and protein. Bananas and chocolate chips provide sweetness without overpowering the peanut butter taste.

gluten-free | high protein | quick & simple | yield: 2 servings

¾ cup (180 ml) plain nonfat Greek yogurt

1 frozen banana, chopped

1 tbsp (16 g) unsweetened creamy peanut butter

2 tbsp (15 g) peanut flour

2 tbsp (22 g) semi-sweet chocolate chips

To a blender or food processor, add the Greek yogurt, frozen banana chunks, peanut butter, and peanut flour and blend until smooth, about 30 seconds.

Stir in the chocolate chips by hand or on the machine's lowest setting for 5 seconds.

Enjoy immediately or store in the freezer for up to 1 month. If freezing, put the frozen yogurt in a parchment-lined loaf pan. Let it sit at room temperature for about 30 minutes before scooping with an ice cream scooper to serve.

> TIP: You can typically find peanut flour, sometimes called powdered peanut butter, either in the baking aisle or with the other peanut butter jars in your local grocery store.

Nutrition Info (Serving size: ½ recipe): Calories: 254, Total Fat: 10 g, Saturated Fat: 4 g, Total Carbohydrates: 29 g, Sugar: 17 g, Fiber: 4 g, Sodium: 86 mg, Protein: 15 g

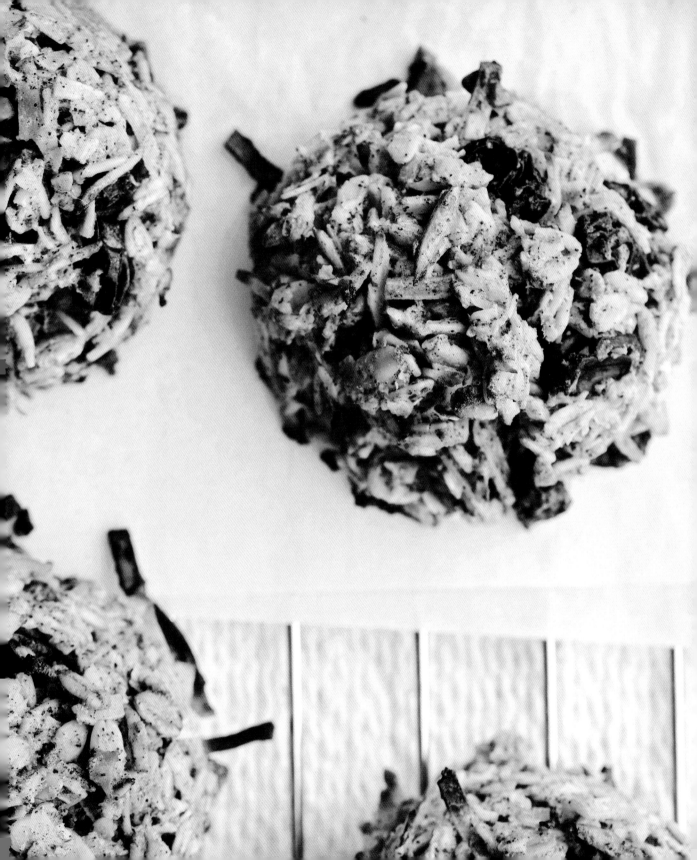

no-added-sugar
sweet treats

Added sugar seems to be gaining a lot of attention in recent years. And rightfully so. But, probably not for the reason you're thinking.

Many people think that naturally occurring sugar is somehow better for you than added sugar. But it's not. Our bodies actually react to them the same way. What is different is what comes along with those naturally occurring sugars.

The recipes in this chapter are sweetened naturally with fruit, milk, and grains. The natural sugar found in fruit, milk, and grains also comes with fiber, vitamins, minerals, and antioxidants. Added sugar doesn't come with those other things. It's just sugar. So, there is an argument to be made that if we're going to sweeten something up, why not use a naturally occurring source and get some additional nutritional benefits along with it?

For example, the Medjool dates in our Pecan Pie Protein Balls (page 140) are a great way to sweeten things up and also provide a rich source of minerals and fiber. Or maybe you're in the mood for a Banana Nut Mug Muffin (page 151), sweetened only with bananas. Bananas offer fiber, potassium, and vitamins!

pecan pie protein balls

With 5 grams of protein in each pecan pie–inspired protein ball, you'll be wondering how you made it this long without this recipe! The fat, fiber, and protein from hemp seeds, flax seeds, and pecans all combine together perfectly into your new favorite sweet treat!

dairy-free | gluten-free | high protein | no added sugar | yield: 12 protein balls

¼ cup (28 g) flax seeds, ground

¼ cup (40 g) hemp hearts, ground

¼ tsp ground cinnamon

Pinch of sea salt

¾ cup (82 g) raw pecan pieces

4 Medjool dates, pitted

½ cup (129 g) unsweetened almond butter

1 tsp vanilla extract

To the bowl of a food processor, add your ground flax seeds, ground hemp hearts, cinnamon, and sea salt. Pulse a few times to get them mixed up.

Then add in your pecan pieces and process them for 15 to 20 seconds, or until they are almost completely ground up.

Next, add in your dates, almond butter, and vanilla extract. Process the mixture again for about 60 seconds, until a thick dough has formed. Refrigerate the dough for 1 hour or longer.

Carefully scoop out the dough and roll it into balls, dividing it into 12 protein balls.

Store your protein balls in the freezer for up to 3 months.

TIPS: You can buy flax seeds and hemp hearts already ground up from your local grocery store, or use a small coffee grinder at home to grind them yourself.

If you're using a food processor to make these protein balls, I recommend using one with a 9 cup (2.1 L) bowl or larger.

Nutrition Info (Serving size: 1 protein ball): Calories: 180, Total Fat: 14 g, Saturated Fat: 1 g, Total Carbohydrates: 13 g, Sugar: 6 g, Fiber: 3 g, Sodium: 14 mg, Protein: 5 g

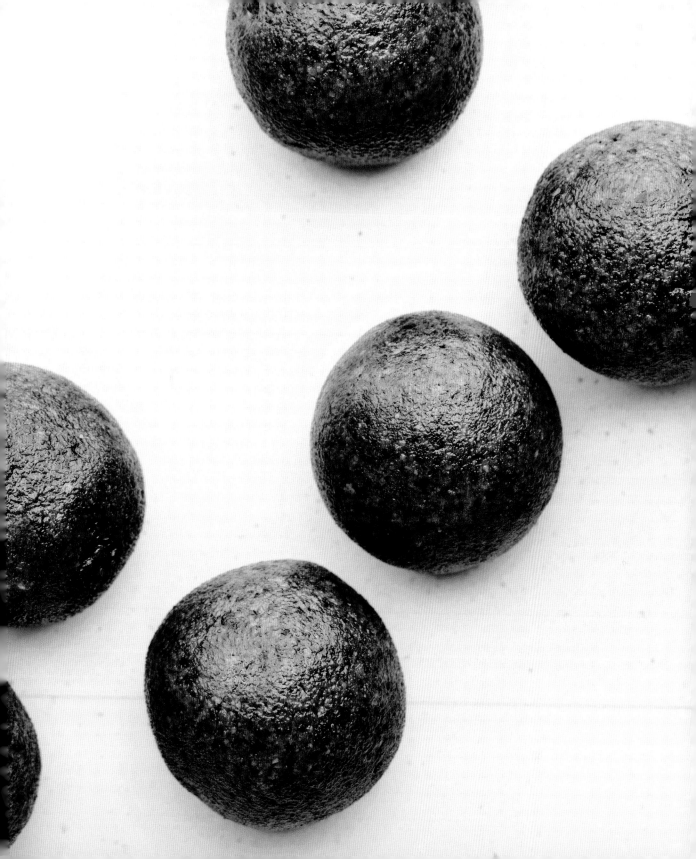

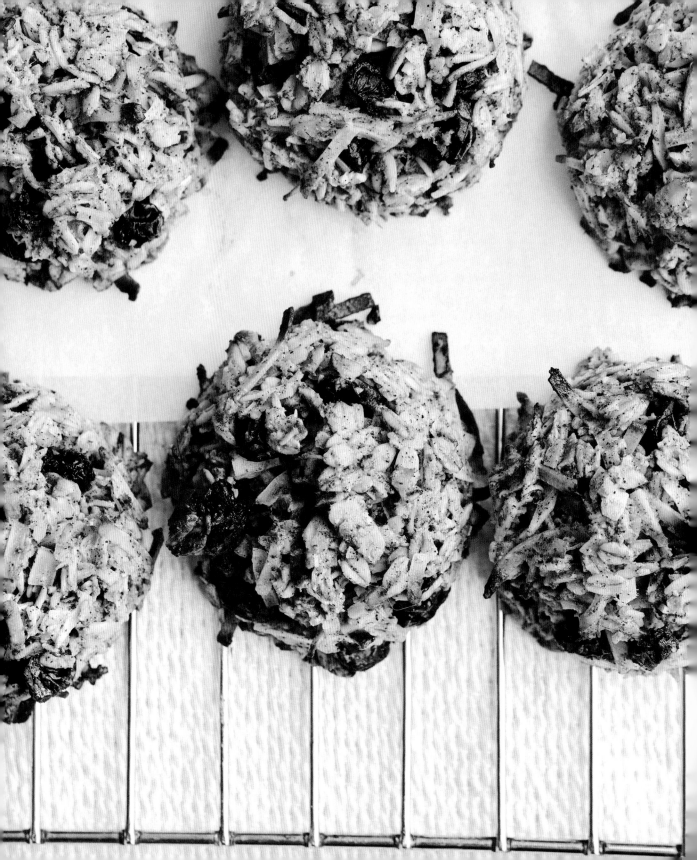

oatmeal raisin snowball cookies

Your oatmeal raisin cookie just got a deliciously coconut-inspired upgrade! Only 6 grams of naturally occurring sugar in each cookie means you can rest assured your blood sugars will stay stable.

high protein | no added sugar | quick & simple | yield: 12 cookies

1½ cups (144 g) shredded unsweetened coconut flakes

2 cups (180 g) rolled oats

1 tbsp (8 g) ground cinnamon

4 large eggs (228 g), beaten

¼ cup (60 ml) plain low-fat Greek yogurt

¼ cup (54 g) unrefined coconut oil, melted

2 tsp (10 ml) vanilla extract

2 tsp (10 ml) almond extract

¼ cup (60 ml) unsweetened applesauce

½ cup (73 g) raisins, packed

Preheat your oven to 375°F (191°C). Line a baking sheet with parchment paper and set it aside.

In a medium-sized bowl, mix together the coconut flakes, rolled oats, cinnamon, eggs, Greek yogurt, coconut oil, vanilla extract, almond extract, applesauce, and raisins. The mixture won't look much like a normal cookie dough, and that's okay!

Using an ice cream scoop, scoop up the mixture and press it into the scoop. Gently drop the scoops about 2 inches (5 cm) apart from each other onto the prepared baking sheet.

Bake the cookies for 15 to 20 minutes, until they are golden brown and the tops are crispy.

Remove the cookies from the oven and let them sit for 5 minutes. Then, transfer them to a cooling rack to finish cooling.

Enjoy your cookies warm, or store them in an airtight container unrefrigerated for up to 3 days. Freeze any remaining cookies after 3 days for up to 6 months.

TIP: When scooping the batter into balls, it's going to seem like they'll just fall apart. Use an ice cream scoop and pack each scoop tightly. Drop them onto the pan and when they're done baking, they'll gel together perfectly!

Nutrition Info (Serving size: 1 cookie): Calories: 178, Total Fat: 11 g, Saturated Fat: 8 g, Total Carbohydrates: 17 g, Sugar: 6 g, Fiber: 3 g, Sodium: 30 mg, Protein: 5 g

chocolate peanut butter stuffed dates

Medjool dates make the perfect base for this chocolate–peanut butter combo. They have a rich, caramel flavor, contain no added sugar, and are packed with fiber. This recipe also uses one of my favorite ways to add sweetness without sugar: extracts!

dairy-free | gluten-free | quick & simple | no added sugar | yield: 24 pieces

2 oz (56 g) unsweetened chocolate (100% cocoa)

1 tbsp (14 g) refined coconut oil

1 tsp almond extract

24 Medjool dates, pitted and sliced in half

½ cup (129 g) unsweetened peanut butter

First get your baking sheet, line it with parchment paper, and set it aside.

In a microwave-safe bowl, melt your unsweetened chocolate and coconut oil according to the chocolate package instructions. Once melted, carefully stir in the almond extract until you have a smooth mixture. Set the chocolate aside.

Then, stuff each date half with 1 teaspoon of peanut butter. Dip the stuffed date in the melted chocolate mixture and place it on the parchment-lined baking sheet.

Set the dates in the freezer for 15 to 20 minutes. Serve immediately or transfer to a storage container and place it in the refrigerator to store until you're ready to eat them.

Store your dates in the refrigerator in a sealed container for 2 to 3 weeks, or in the freezer for up to 3 months.

TIP: Feel free to substitute any nut butter of choice.

Nutrition Info (Serving size: 2 pieces): Calories: 222, Total Fat: 9 g, Saturated Fat: 4 g, Total Carbohydrates: 34 g, Sugar: 26 g, Fiber: 4 g, Sodium: 2 mg, Protein: 4 g

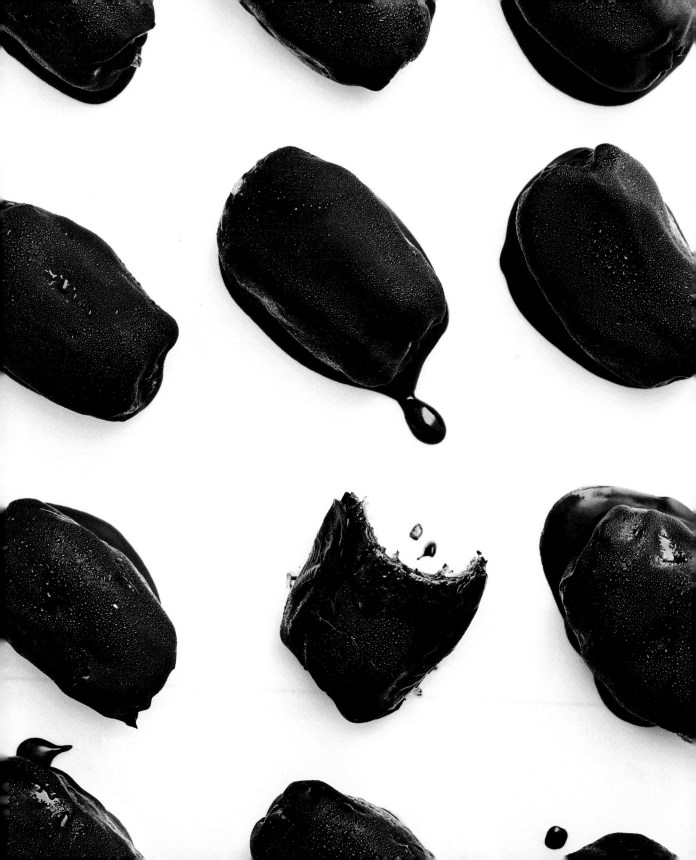

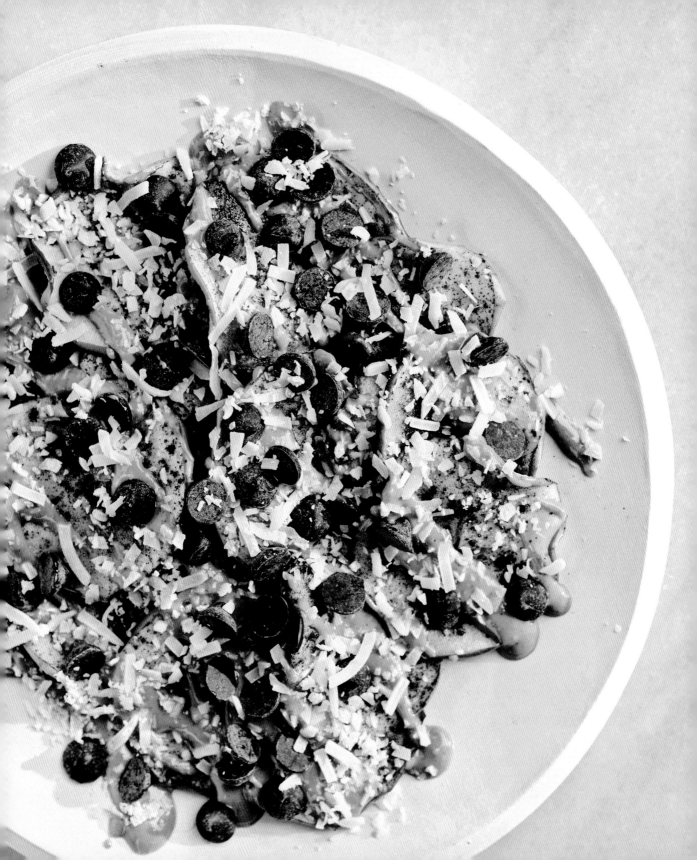

apple dessert nachos

I almost feel guilty for calling this a recipe because it's so simple. Apples are naturally rich in fiber and sweetness, and when we add some plant-based fats from peanut butter and coconut, we've got the perfect formula for stable blood sugars and no added sugar!

dairy-free | gluten-free | high fiber | no added sugar | quick & simple | yield: 2 servings

1 small Fuji apple (129 g)

Cooking oil spray

½ tsp ground cinnamon

1 tbsp (16 g) unsweetened peanut butter

1 tbsp (6 g) unsweetened coconut flakes

2 tbsp (22 g) no-added-sugar chocolate chips

Preheat your oven to 400°F (201°C). Line a baking sheet with parchment paper and set it aside. Wash and dry your apple, and then cut it horizontally into thin round circles. Remove the seeds as you get to them while slicing.

Arrange the apple slices on the prepared baking sheet. Spray the apple slices with your cooking spray, and sprinkle the cinnamon over the apple slices. Place them in the oven for 10 to 12 minutes, until they are somewhat fork tender but have a slight crisp left to them. (You should also be able to hear them sizzling quite well!)

Let the apple slices cool, then arrange them on a plate and drizzle the peanut butter on top. Then, sprinkle your coconut flakes and chocolate chips on.

These don't store long-term very well, so eat up right after you serve them!

TIP: I love Fuji apples for how sweet they taste, but you can use your favorite kind of apple too!

Nutrition Info (Serving size: ½ apple nacho plate): Calories: 166, Total Fat: 10 g, Saturated Fat: 5 g, Total Carbohydrates: 22 g, Sugar: 10 g, Fiber: 7 g, Sodium: 33 mg, Protein: 3 g

easy rainbow fruit pizza

Traditional fruit pizza recipes feature sugar cookie dough as a crust and are loaded with a high-sugar fruit dip as a sauce. But you simply don't need all that added sugar to enjoy a great fruit pizza! Here I'm using a simple, nutrient-dense crust (sweetened with dates), and all we need is plain Greek yogurt and some lemon zest for the perfect "sauce"!

high protein | no added sugar | quick & simple | yield: 12 servings

2 cups (190 g) almond flour

½ cup (45 g) oats, ground

4 Medjool dates, pitted

¼ cup (54 g) coconut oil, melted

1 large egg (57 g)

½ tsp almond extract

½ tsp vanilla extract

½ cup (120 ml) plain low-fat Greek yogurt, divided

½ tbsp (3 g) lemon zest

5–6 large strawberries (60 g), sliced thin

2 mandarin oranges (176 g), peeled and separated

¼ cup (41 g) sliced pineapple

2 kiwi fruit (138 g), peeled and sliced

¼ cup (37 g) blueberries

Preheat your oven to 350°F (177°C). Cut a circle of parchment paper to fit the bottom of an 8- or 9-inch (20- or 23-cm) round cake pan and place it in the pan. Set the prepared pan aside.

Using a food processor or blender, combine all of your almond flour, oats, dates, coconut oil, egg, almond extract, and vanilla extract and blend until a dough forms. Spread the batter into the prepared pan. Bake the fruit pizza crust for 20 to 22 minutes, or until the edges are browned.

Remove the crust from the oven and let it cool until the pan is safe to handle without burning your hands. Turn the pan upside down and the crust should fall right out. (You may need to run a knife around the edges before doing this.) Remove the parchment paper and turn the crust back over.

Once it's completely cooled, top the crust with the plain Greek yogurt. (Spread it out like you would pizza sauce on a pizza.) Sprinkle the lemon zest on top of the Greek yogurt.

Then, add your sliced strawberries, orange slices, sliced pineapple, sliced kiwi, and blueberries on top!

The assembled pizza won't keep well, but the crust can be made ahead of time and stored in the refrigerator for up to 1 week or frozen for up to 6 months.

TIP: If you want to kick up the flavor even more without adding any additional sugar, top the Greek yogurt layer with some orange zest as well!

Nutrition Info (Serving size: ¹⁄₁₂ of pizza): Calories: 211, Total Fat: 15 g, Saturated Fat: 5 g, Total Carbohydrates: 17 g, Sugar: 8 g, Fiber: 4 g, Sodium: 12 mg, Protein: 6 g

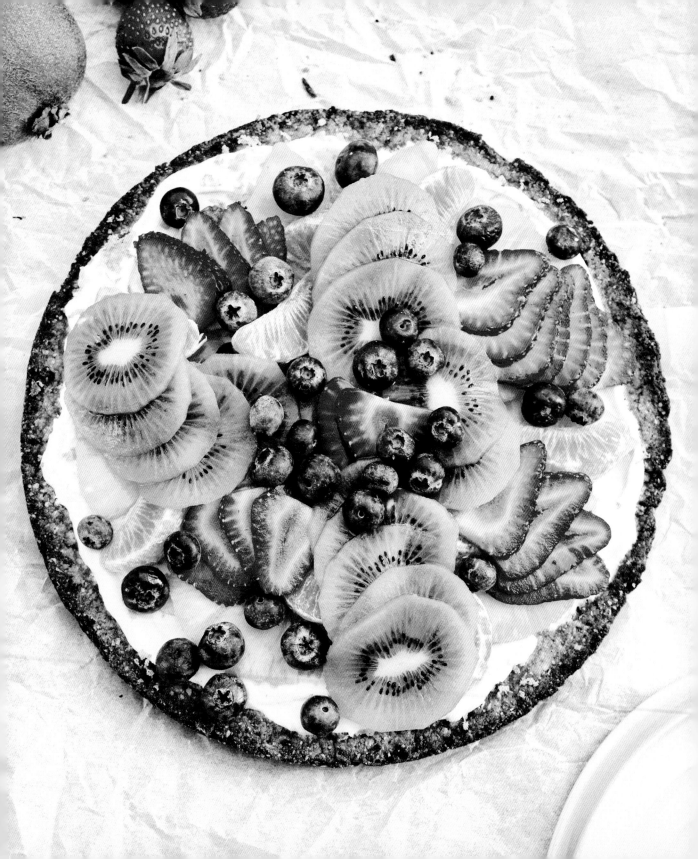

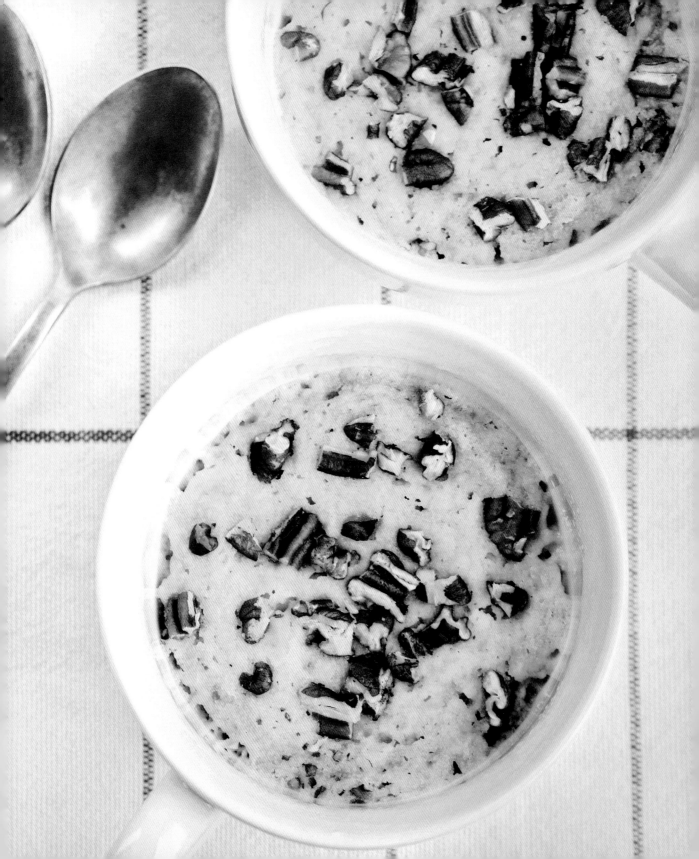

banana nut mug muffin

Wondering what to do with that random overripe banana sitting on your counter? Well, this is the recipe for you! Turn that banana into the most blood sugar–friendly, high-fiber, high-protein treat in under 5 minutes with the recipe below!

dairy-free | gluten-free | high fiber | high protein | quick & simple | no added sugar | yield: 2 mug muffins

1 small ripe banana, mashed

2 tbsp (30 ml) unsweetened almond milk

½ cup (48 g) almond flour

Pinch of sea salt

½ tsp baking powder

½ tsp vanilla extract

1 tbsp (7 g) pecan pieces

Grease the inside of two small microwave-safe coffee mugs. In a small bowl, whisk the mashed banana, almond milk, almond flour, sea salt, baking powder, and vanilla extract thoroughly to combine. Divide the batter evenly into your greased coffee mugs.

Next, sprinkle the pecan pieces on top of each mug.

Place the coffee mugs in the microwave for 2 to 3 minutes. You'll know they're done when you see that they have risen and the centers are no longer wet. Let the muffins cool in the coffee mugs for about 2 minutes before handling.

Eat and enjoy straight from the mug, or transfer them out of the coffee mugs and store them in a sealed container on the counter for up to 2 days.

TIP: Microwave oven cooking times vary so make sure to keep an eye on your mug cake to know when it is done. If you discover your mug muffin isn't cooked all the way through, just pop it back in the microwave for an additional 30 to 60 seconds.

Nutrition Info (Serving size: 1 mug muffin): Calories: 225, Total Fat: 14 g, Saturated Fat: 1 g, Total Carbohydrates: 19 g, Sugar: 7 g, Fiber: 5 g, Sodium: 85 mg, Protein: 8 g

cinnamon roll snack bites

Nothing beats a cinnamon roll fresh out of the oven in the morning (seriously, make sure to try The Easiest Healthy Cinnamon Rolls [page 84]), but these cinnamon roll snack bites come in a pretty close second! Since there's no added sugar, plus 3 grams of protein and 2 grams of fiber in each bite, you can rest assured your blood sugars will be stable and your taste buds will be happy!

dairy-free | no added sugar | yield: 12 snack bites

½ cup (129 g) almond butter

¼ cup (60 ml) unsweetened applesauce

½ tsp vanilla extract

½ cup (48 g) almond flour

½ cup (45 g) rolled oats

1 tsp ground cinnamon

CINNAMON "SUGAR" COATING (OPTIONAL)

1 tsp ground cinnamon

7–8 packets (25 g) of your favorite zero-sugar sweetener (stevia, monk fruit extract, etc.)

In a bowl, thoroughly mix together your almond butter, applesauce, vanilla extract, almond flour, oats, and cinnamon until a dough forms. Place the dough in the refrigerator for 1 to 2 hours.

Once chilled, remove the dough from the refrigerator and roll it into 12 balls.

Now, if you want to add the cinnamon "sugar" coating, combine the cinnamon and your packets of zero-sugar sweetener in a small bowl. Roll each snack bite in the cinnamon mixture to thoroughly coat it and you're done!

Store your snack bites in the refrigerator in a sealed container for up to 2 weeks. You can also freeze these snack bites for up to 6 months.

TIP: If you prefer for your snack bites to be a uniform texture, grind your oats up before mixing them into your dough.

Nutrition Info (Serving size: 1 snack bite): Calories: 105, Total Fat: 8 g, Saturated Fat: 1 g, Total Carbohydrates: 6 g, Sugar: 1 g, Fiber: 2 g, Sodium: 1 mg, Protein: 3 g

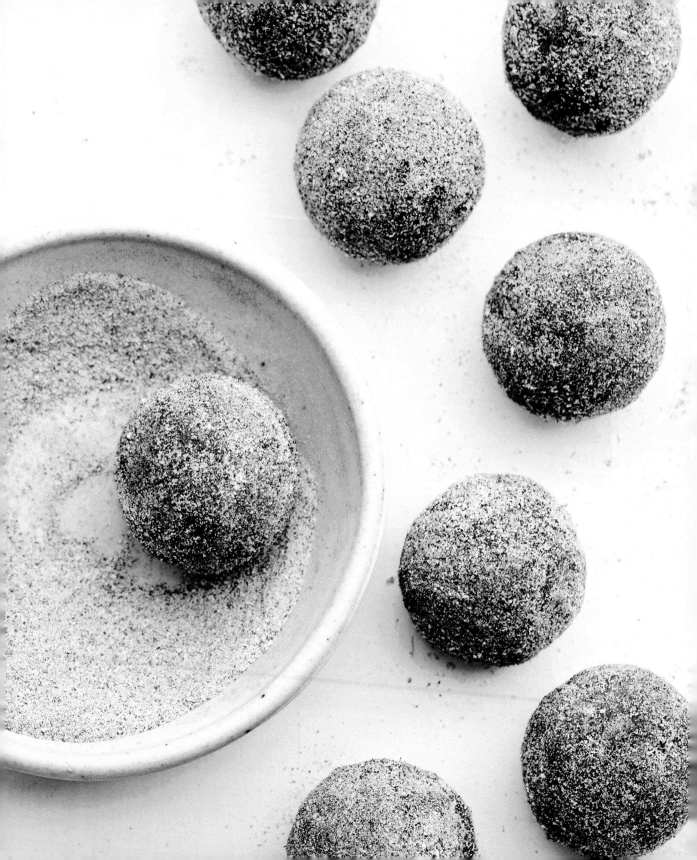

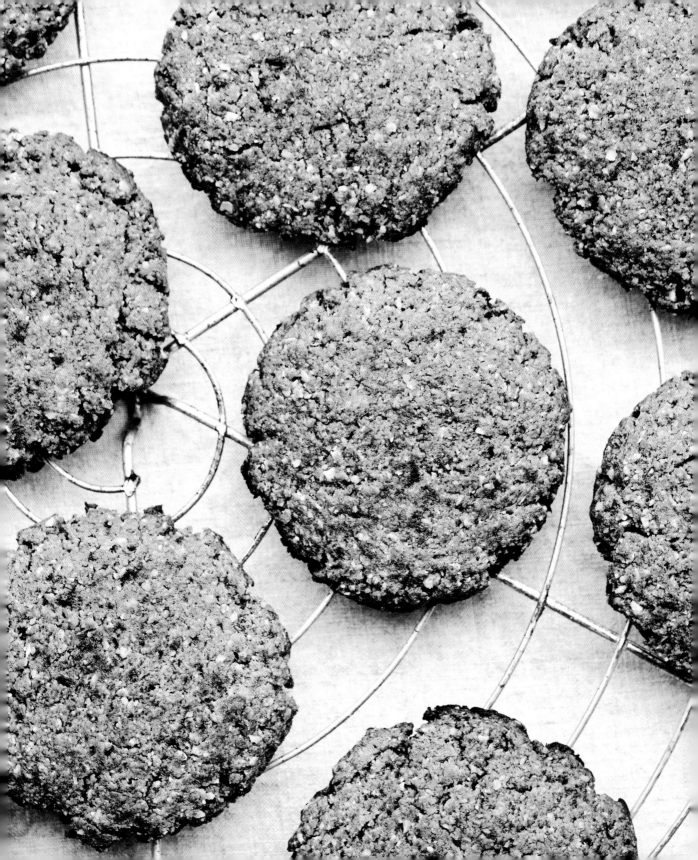

peanut butter date cookies

These cookies could not get any simpler or more delicious. With 5 grams of protein in just one cookie, they're the perfect way to keep blood sugars stable so you can power through your day!

dairy-free | high protein | no added sugar | quick & simple | yield: 18 cookies

1 cup (90 g) rolled oats

1 tsp cinnamon

½ cup (48 g) almond flour

½ tsp baking soda

¾ cup (194 g) unsweetened peanut butter

10 Medjool dates, pitted

1 large egg (57 g)

½ tsp vanilla extract

2 tbsp (30 ml) water

Preheat your oven to 350°F (177°C) and line a baking sheet with parchment paper. Set the baking sheet aside.

In the bowl of a food processor, add the oats, cinnamon, almond flour, and baking soda and process until they form a uniform powder. This should only take 10 to 15 seconds. Next, add in the peanut butter, dates, egg, vanilla extract, and water. Process until a dough forms, about 60 seconds.

Remove the dough from the food processor and divide it evenly into 18 dough balls. Place the dough balls 1½ to 2 inches (4 to 5 cm) apart on the parchment-lined pan, and press them flat until they're about 2 inches (5 cm) across. Place the pan in the oven and bake for 12 to 15 minutes, or until they start to firm up and lift off the parchment paper easily.

Remove the cookies from the oven and transfer them to a cooling rack.

Store your cookies in an airtight container on the counter for up to 5 days. You can also freeze them in a sealed container for up to 6 months.

TIPS: If the dough doesn't start to clump together or appears too dry in the food processor, add some water a ½ tablespoon (8 ml) at a time until a dough ball starts to form.

Nutrition Info (Serving size: 1 cookie): Calories: 140, Total Fat: 7 g, Saturated Fat: 1 g, Total Carbohydrates: 16 g, Sugar: 10 g, Fiber: 2 g, Sodium: 41 mg, Protein: 5 g

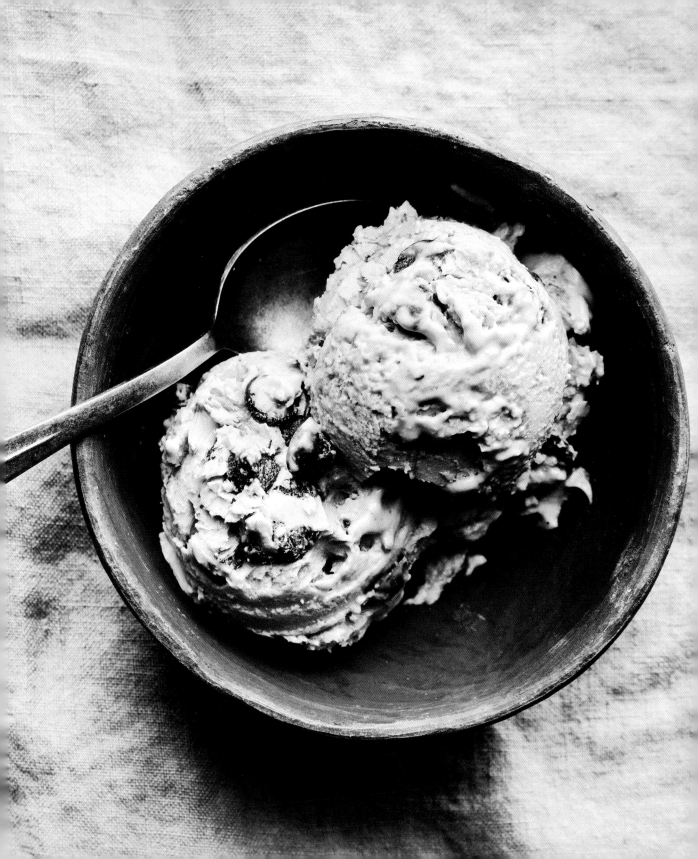

acknowledgments

There are many aspects of my career that I never saw coming, but writing cookbooks is something I've dreamed about since I was a little girl. I want to thank the following people for helping my dreams come true . . .

My grandmothers, for showing me from an early age that food is meant to be joyful!

My parents, for always encouraging me and raising me to know that diabetes would never stand in the way of accomplishing my goals.

Danielle Fineberg, this book would not exist without you! Thank you for all of your recipe testing, fine-tuning, and helping to make this book exactly what I envisioned it to be.

The Page Street Publishing team, for believing in me yet again!

Constance Mariena, your ability to bring recipes to life in photos is unmatched . . . This book is truly a work of art because of you!

Jenny Noonan and Allie Saxton, thank you for baking up a storm and helping test these recipes in the middle of one of the hottest summers ever.

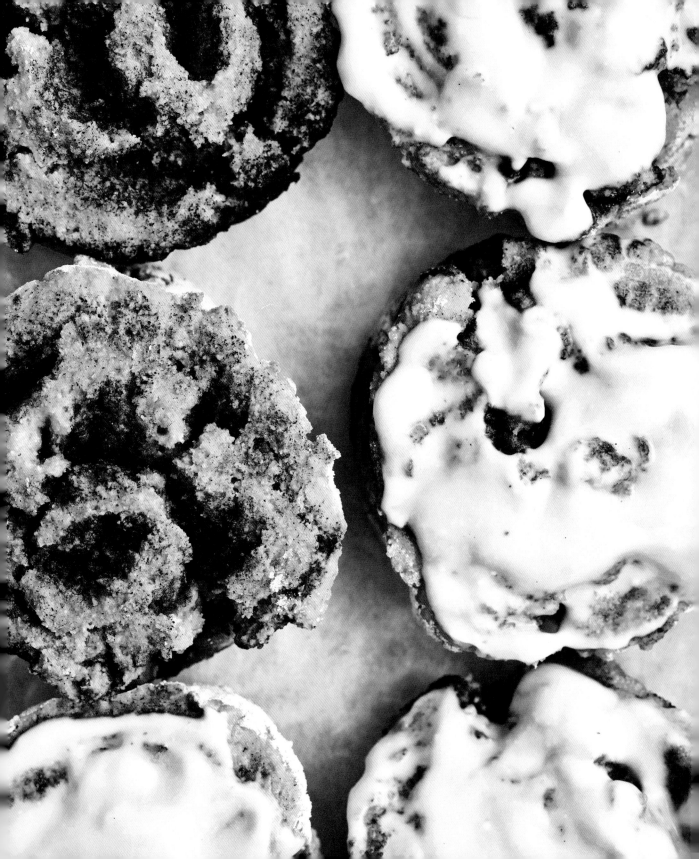

about the author

Mary Ellen Phipps is the founder, author, and registered dietitian behind Milk & Honey Nutrition®. Mary Ellen has been living with type 1 diabetes since she was five years old, and she knows firsthand the impact food has on how we think, feel, act, and move. She strives to make food easy and fun for people with diabetes. She uses both her professional expertise and personal experience to reduce stress and fear around food and to help people find joy in the kitchen again. You can connect with her at milkandhoneynutrition.com.

Mary Ellen is the bestselling author of *The Easy Diabetes Cookbook*, and is also a contributing writer, recipe developer, and content expert for several leading health and wellness organizations. You can find her frequently on Houston-area TV stations educating audiences on food, nutrition, and joyful eating. She received a Bachelor of Science degree in Nutritional Sciences from Baylor University and a Master of Public Health degree in Epidemiology from the University of Texas School of Public Health.

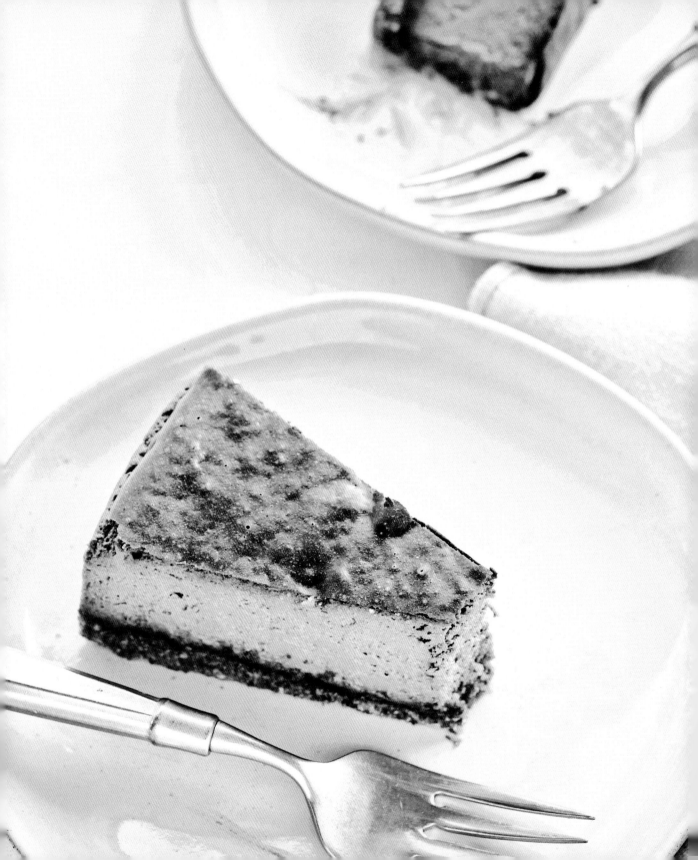

index